Educating the Dentist of the Future

Educating the Dentist of the Future:

THE PENNSYLVANIA EXPERIMENT

D. Walter Cohen, D.D.S.
Patricia P. Cormier, Ed.D.
Joanne L. Cohen, A.B.

University of Pennsylvania Press • Philadelphia

This work was published with the support of the Pew Memorial Trust.

Library of Congress Cataloging in Publication Data

Cohen, D. Walter (David Walter), 1926–
  Educating the dentist of the future.

  Bibliography: p.
  1. Dentistry—Study in teaching—Pennsylvania.
I. Cormier, Patricia P., 1939– .   II. Cohen, Joanne L.
III. Title.
RD96.P4C65   1985   617.6'007'1174811   84–19602
ISBN 0–8122–7947–6

Printed in the United States of America

Contents

List of Figures

List of Tables

To
Robert G. Dunlop and *Robert I. Smith,*
whose confidence and vision
made this experiment possible, and to the
faculty and students
who made it a success

Acknowledgments

The support and assistance that the authors received in writing this volume are testimony to the positive feelings engendered by the Pennsylvania Experiment. Many members of the University of Pennsylvania dental community, eager to see the story of the experiment appear in print and the results made public, contributed time and energy to this project. Most of the text is based on personal interviews with these persons. The authors wish to acknowledge the invaluable assistance of Morton Amsterdam, Paul Berson, Meredith Bogert, Daniel Casullo, Deborah Diserens, James Galbally, Jeffrey Garber, Ali Geranmayeh, Carolyn Locke, Stephen Locke, Edward Lusk, Herbert Myers, Cathy Schifter, Robert Tisot, Stephen Wotman, and Robert Zemsky.

A large portion of this text is drawn from the Busch Center Report on the educational, financial, and managerial dimensions of the Pennsylvania Experiment. Chapters 6 and 7 are excerpted directly from this report, which was largely the work of three principal members of the Busch Center: Jamshid Gharajedaghia, Edward Lusk, and Ali Geranmayeh. Their contributions as outside evaluators of the Pennsylvania Experiment and as managerial consultants added a critically important dimension to the experiment.

Neither this book nor the experiment could ever have occurred without the extremely generous support of the Pew Memorial Trust administered by the Glenmede Trust Company. Through the Trust's donations the Pennsylvania Experiment was translated from a dream on paper to a living experiment in dental education. The Pew Memorial Trust also financed publication of this book so that the results of the experiment can be shared with the health care community. The University of Pennsylvania School of Dental Medicine owes a tremendous debt to the Glenmede Trust Company, and we would like to express here our profound gratitude for its unfailing generosity and support of the future of dental education at Pennsylvania.

Dean Jan Lindhe reviewed all of the material available on the Pennsylvania Experiment before he accepted the position of Dean of the University of Pennsylvania School of Dental Medicine. His insight into the depth and value of this educational research is greatly appreciated.

In addition, we would like to thank the following people for their clerical and technical contributions to this book: Allan Hoffman, Catherine Redden, Marion Kane, Elaine Reeder, Carol Wanamaker, Gloria Weagly, and Sheri Wingert.

The experiment was the combined effort of many students, faculty, staff members, and administrators. We have acknowledged their invaluable contributions to the experiment by listing their names in the appendixes to the book. We would like to recognize especially the University of Pennsylvania and its principal administrators at the time of the experiment: Presidents Martin Meyerson and Sheldon Hackney, Vice-President for Health Affairs Thomas Langfitt, and Provosts Vartan Gregorian and Thomas Ehrlich, for providing a supportive environment which encouraged experimentation and innovation.

The Pennsylvania Experiment: Educating the Dentist of the Future

Dental education faces tremendous challenges in this era, which many educators and practitioners have called one of crisis and retrenchment. Constrained by severe financial limitations, dental schools must continue to prepare students for their roles as the professionals of the future. This task is especially difficult because the oral health needs of the population have changed dramatically in the past twenty years, and the professional environment in which the graduate will function is barely recognizable when compared with that of twenty years ago. The challenge to dental education has never been greater; clearly, the solutions that emerge will have a significant impact on the dental profession and on the oral health of the population during the remainder of this century.

Financial Issues in Dental Education

The financial situation in dental education has become very difficult in recent years. This situation is closely linked to health manpower planning. During the 1970s, dental schools relied heavily on capitation (systematic subsidization of dental education by the federal government) as a source of funding. The capitation program was based on predictions of an imminent shortage of health professionals. Capitation funding matched a certain percentage of students' tuition monies, provided that a sufficient number of students were enrolled. In 1979, however, with warnings of a possible oversupply of health professionals, and in an era of unrelenting inflation and a "no-growth" economy, the government discontinued capitation.

At the same time, dental schools, along with most areas of higher education, have been suffering from reductions in private and state funding. The financial situation in dental education, however, is compounded by several other problems that are unique to the profession. Since 1975, there has been a steady decline in the number of students applying to dental schools. This decline is caused by several factors, including a decline in the number of eighteen-to-twenty-four-year-olds in the population and perceptions by potential students that dental education is very costly and that the profession is overcrowded. Schools are now forced to compete for qualified students and for tuition dollars. Many predict that this trend will continue well into the 1990s. Patient pools for student clinics have also decreased in size because of the growth of third-party coverage for dental care, which has enabled many patients to seek treatment from private practitioners rather than student clinics. The combination of these factors has created a grim financial picture in dental education. As Dr. Richard S. MacKenzie stated: "We are now at the initial stages of a no-growth economy, heavier competition for both clinical patients and potential students. . . . What this may mean to dental education is belt-tightening, reduction of dental faculty, perhaps the loss of a few dental schools, and greater competition for financial and patient resources."[1]

Educational Issues in Dental Education

The financial crisis in dental education occurs at a time when dental schools face a unique set of educational challenges as well. The dental profession has undergone complete transformation during the past twenty years; a plethora of new terms such as retail dentistry, health maintenance organizations, third-party carriers, dental hygiene practices, and others are indicators of fundamental changes in what has become a dynamic and complex professional environment.

Twenty years ago the predominant mode of delivery in dentistry was the solo, fee-for-service practice; now alternative forms of financing and delivering care are common. In particular, the group practice has emerged as a desirable form of delivery. In a 1980 survey of United States dental deans, all respondents predicted that in twenty years, 20 to 29 percent of all practices will be group practices.[2] In predicting the future of health care in this country, Dr. Charles Jerge stated: "Solo practice will probably persist indefinitely, although younger practitioners—dental and medical alike—will no doubt gravitate toward group practice and other organizational forms. While the solo practitioner of today will not precipitously disappear, there will likely be a major movement toward relatively small (seven to ten practitioners) private dental group practices as well as considerable participation on the part of dentists in community health centers, health maintenance organizations (HMOs), community hospitals, and other health care service and educational institutions."[3]

The use of multihanded, sit-down dentistry and expanded-function dental auxiliaries also has gained increased acceptance in dental practice. This trend is likely to continue. Further, most practices now use one or several alternative forms of financing care. As of 1982, approximately 80 million people were covered by some form of dental insurance.[4] The growth of third-party payments and other alternative forms of financing has created an entirely new set of practice management issues for the dental health practitioner. The traditional model of the self-employed dentist has also been modified because of the financial difficulties associated with starting a new practice, many graduates now elect salaried positions.

These major changes in the delivery and financing of care call for a sophisticated, knowledgeable professional, one who is prepared to function within a group setting if she or he chooses, able to deal with the complexities of practice management, and experienced in the most modern techniques of dental care delivery.

At the same time, the epidemiology of the population has changed dramatically, in large measure because of preventive measures. Widespread fluoridation of water supplies and other fluoride modalities have resulted in substantial reductions in the incidence of coronal or primary dental caries in children in many communities. Although the need for restorative services has by no means disappeared, the dental health needs of the population are focused more now in the areas of prevention, periodontics, orthodontics, and endodontics. Also, as life expectancies increase and as the profession attempts to improve access for elderly as well as handicapped patients, more geriatric and medically compromised patients will be seen in dental offices, further altering the composition of the patient population. Dental professionals of the future will need to have increased clinical competence, be able to treat more advanced types of dental disease, and be knowledgeable about patients' overall oral health needs.

The recent phenomenon of oversupply within the profession, resulting in increased competitiveness, adds yet another dimension to a stressful professional environment. The Committee on the Future of Dentistry, commissioned by the American Dental Association (ADA) to predict and make recommendations concerning the future of the profession, concluded that "there is an adequate national supply of dental manpower, and in some regions, an oversupply."[5] Recent developments such as retail dentistry, advertising, and attempts by some dentists to adopt a flashier, more personable image reflect in part this competitive atmosphere. Not only must the dental school graduate be able to deal with the realities of complex practice management issues and a different disease base in the population, but she/he will have to do so within a highly competitive marketplace.

How can dental schools respond to these challenges in the face of severe financial constraints? How can they update and improve their educational programs in an era of reduced fiscal support and a limited pool of applicants? Clearly there is a need for innovative, creative solutions to plan for the future of dental education and the dental profession. As Dr. Frederick M. Parkins stated: "It seems clear that dental education is in a period of transition and retrenchment, a period of transition from relatively extensive federal support

to little or no support, and a period of retrenchment from fairly abundant resources to resources that are barely adequate to meet the minimum needs of
the educational programs. . . . Fundamental changes are taking place and, for
some, it could mean years of crisis. Ultimately, I believe that dental education
will be judged by its ability to react to the crisis in a positive way—by using
the opportunities to alter priorities and to make the program changes needed
for operating within available resources, while still preparing future dentists
for new modes of practice."[6]

The Pennsylvania Experiment

From 1979 to 1982, two of the authors conducted a pilot program at the University of Pennsylvania School of Dental Medicine to study an alternative to
the current educational and financial structure of dental education. Known as
the Pennsylvania Experiment, this study attempted to address many of these
financial and educational issues, testing a program designed to educate the
dentist of the future in a financially viable way.

The Pennsylvania Experiment was funded by a three-year grant from the Pew
Memorial Trust of the Glenmede Trust Company. A small group of faculty,
students, and administrators within the University of Pennsylvania School of
Dental Medicine participated in a separate curriculum and program of education during academic years 1979–80, 1980–81, and 1981–82. The experiment
centered around the preceptor model of education, in which predoctoral students learned dentistry by observing faculty members in practice and then
performing the techniques they had witnessed. Students had their entire clinical education within either a small clinical setting featuring extended
teaching-practice roles by faculty members (Model A); or a faculty-based private group practice (Model B). These settings were alternatives to the large
clinical setting of the dental school, in which all other students received their
clinical education. Other alterations in the dental school curriculum included
an integrated preclinical laboratory course, greater coordination between preclinical and clinical learning, a comprehensive clinical setting that eliminated
rotations into specialty clinics by bringing specialists together in one setting
with generalist faculty, new courses in areas such as human behavior and practice management, and, finally, a fifth-year general dentistry program as a mandatory component of the D.M.D. curriculum.

FINANCIAL ASPECTS OF THE PENNSYLVANIA EXPERIMENT
The Pennsylvania Experiment addressed several of the key financial issues in-
herent in dental education today. First, it tested the use of a faculty-based pri-

vate practice that also served as an educational unit for students. The faculty practice offers a source of income for dental schools at a time when outside funding is scarce. Such practices have the potential not only to assume the cost of faculty salaries but also to generate surplus income for the school. The Pennsylvania Experiment explored this alternative fully, determining the managerial and financial ingredients that constitute a successful faculty-based practice/educational unit.

Also central to the new program was a reduction in class size. Like the faculty practice, this measure was seen as necessary to create a program of academic excellence; it is also a timely solution to current fiscal realities. Concerns about oversupply in the profession and shrinking applicant pools make reduced class sizes inevitable. The Committee on the Future of Dentistry stated: "With the current and projected demand for dental services, it appears that the trend toward a reduction in the number of dentists being trained is in the best interest of the public in conserving resources."[7]

The issue of shrinking patient pools for student clinics was also addressed by the experiment. The faculty-based private practice/educational unit is an ideal solution to this problem. Patients opting for private treatment have expressed a willingness to be treated by students if their care is supervised by faculty-providers. Therefore, students can maintain a healthy patient base by practicing within a faculty practice setting.

Yet another financial issue in dental education addressed by the experiment was the fifth-year residency program. Both the American Association of Dental Schools and the American Dental Association have stressed the importance of residency programs in dental education; many have predicted that eventually the fifth year will become a mandatory part of dental education. (It is already mandatory in Sweden.) Yet in a recent conference on graduate dental education, the financial viability of such programs was cited as a major unsolved problem.[8] The Pennsylvania Experiment attempted to produce a financially self-sustaining residency program.

EDUCATIONAL ASPECTS OF THE EXPERIMENT

Although the Pennsylvania Experiment addressed current financial issues, its primary aim was to improve the education of the dental professional. In formulating the new program, the originators of the experiment asked one fundamental question: What should the dental professional of the future be, and how can we best prepare students for this role? All planning efforts revolved around the answer to this question.

The members of the committee that planned the experiment concluded that the dentist of the future will be a highly competent generalist, that is, a general practitioner of dentistry with extended clinical competence and skills, able to perform many of the procedures currently referred to specialists, and concerned with prevention, orthodontics, periodontics, and endodontics as well as restorative services. She/he will function as a member of a health care team, coordinating care and planning the overall oral health needs of the patient, referring advanced cases of dental disease to specialists when necessary, and using expanded-function dental auxiliaries for basic dental procedures.

Epidemiologic changes in the population during the past twenty years have created the need for a new type of practitioner. With a dramatic reduction in coronal caries in children and a comparable reduction in the demand for restorative services, the attention of practitioners should emphasize prevention and periodontal, orthodontic, and endodontic care. The survey of dental deans previously cited points toward a difference in the mix of services that should be offered during the next twenty to twenty-five years, with the majority suggesting an increase in the amount of time spent on periodontics and orthodontics.[9] Currently, general practitioners spend minimal time, less than 3 percent according to 1979 statistics, on the periodontal and orthodontic needs of the population.[10] Many patients who have received care on a regular basis later discover that they are suffering from periodontal disease.

A reorganization of the mix of services offered by general practitioners is clearly necessary, with the generalist performing the procedures currently performed by the specialist and referring cases to the specialist based on knowledge of the patients' overall needs. Such a reorganization will meet the dental health needs of the population in the most efficient means possible.

This shift in treatment patterns also may prevent the profession from becoming further specialized and fragmented. As Dr. Morton Amsterdam stated: "Ultimately, we have become so specialized that even the various specialties cannot communicate, and there is no one to coordinate their efforts."[11] The well-educated generalist should assume the role of coordinator of patient care, integrating the efforts of the various specialties. Along this line, the Committee on the Future of Dentistry reported, "The Committee believes that a higher ratio [of specialists] is not in the best interest of the public. The Study of Graduate Medical Education by the National Advisory Committee to the Secretary of the United States Department of Health and Human Services clearly indicates the adverse effects to the public of an oversupply of medical specialists. The American Association of Dental School–sponsored study, *Advanced Dental Education: Recommendations for the 80's*, identified the trend toward increased specialty manpower as a serious potential problem. The Committee . . . is concerned that a continued overproduction in selected specialty areas will adversely affect the efficient delivery of dental care." The report concluded: "The need for selected specialty services will diminish sharply during the next twenty years. While there will be a continuing need for highly competent specialty practitioners, the scope of practice in some specialty areas is too limited to flourish."[12] The committee recommended extended clinical competence by the general practitioner as a solution.

Accordingly, the Pennsylvania Experiment was designed to produce a highly competent generalist. This goal was accomplished in several ways. First, the experiment facilitated an integrated approach to dentistry by eliminating the fragmentation of clinical education into specialty departments. Although the goal of predoctoral dental education is to produce a generalist, students are usually educated in up to nine different specialty departments in an approach to dentistry that becomes fragmented and compartmentalized. They learn endodontics in the endodontics department, periodontics in the periodontics department, and so on, rotating from clinic to clinic with their patients. Ironically, the goal of this fragmented approach is to produce a generalist; when students graduate they will practice all aspects of general dentistry in one setting. By contrast, in the experiment, students received all of their clinical education in one integrated setting (with the exception of one or two rotations), and they were taught by generalists and specialists functioning together to provide high-quality patient care.

In dental schools the preclinical and clinical education of students are generally fragmented. Students usually spend two years in preclinical laboratories before they see techniques performed on patients in the clinical environment. By contrast, in the experiment students were exposed to clinical practice during their first semester of dental school, when they entered the clinical environment as dental assistants. Furthermore, their preclinical learning took place directly adjacent to the clinical setting of Model A, further integrating preclinical and clinical learning.

In addition, students were provided with extended clinical skills through the fifth-year residency program to enable them to acquire the skills of a highly competent generalist. (The residency program was subsequently accredited as an advanced general dentistry program; however, the word "residency" refers to the fifth-year program throughout the experiment.) This program featured advanced didactic and clinical training in all the specialties as well as material on care of the medically compromised patient, peer review, practice management, teaching skills, communication skills, and rotation to hospital settings. Students in the Model B faculty practice were provided with a role model of faculty practitioners functioning as expert generalists; the faculty members in the program were master clinicians with extended competence in at least one specialty area. Students in Model A also received increased exposure to generalist faculty members performing hands-on dentistry.

As discussed above, the dentist of the future will be required to understand the realities of practice management in the 1980s and 1990s. Practice management is acknowledged by many to be grossly underrepresented in the dental school curriculum; students often report after graduation that they were inadequately prepared in this area. In the Pennsylvania Experiment, students within both Models A and B received experience in the realities of practice management. Students in Model B were coproviders in a group practice, thus learning directly the ramifications of dental insurance, appointment scheduling, and the like. In addition, a didactic course in practice management was included in the experimental program.

Although some students in the future will elect solo private practice, graduates must be prepared to function collaboratively in a group practice. Unfortunately, "essentially, dental education has prepared the dental practitioner for solo practice. With rare exception, all of the curriculum and its manner of presentation and acceptance directs a student to solo practice."[13] The dental professional of the future will have to be prepared for the realities of group practice. In the experiment, students in both Models A and B learned collaborative skills as members of dental health teams that included faculty generalists and specialists, residents, students, hygienists, and assistants.

Another feature of the experiment was an emphasis on improving students' interpersonal skills. The first-year curriculum included a human behavior course, supplemented by implicit learning in this area through the presence of faculty role models. Behavioral science courses are often limited in their effectiveness because students are not exposed to faculty actually interacting with patients. As S. R. Dworkin, a behavioral scientist, stated: "Practicing dentists, when they come into the dental clinic as teachers, act as though they were expected to leave behind their repository of information and methods that enable them daily to reduce aversive behavior and facilitate positive oral health behavior in their dental patients."[14]

The Pennsylvania Experiment was also designed to be a humane alternative to many traditional dental school programs. Dental students report that dental school is stressful; the aggravations of large clinical settings often include waiting for supplies in long lines, difficulty in locating faculty members, and other bureaucratic, dehumanizing stresses. The creators of the experiment recognized that environment plays as significant a role in the learning process as many other factors and attempted to create an optimal learning setting for students. Both experimental models were small in size and featured good student-faculty ratios, thereby removing many of the bureaucratic problems of dental education. The student-faculty ratio was created to allow students to work closely with faculty members. Faculty members were able to become familiar with students personally, instructing them on the basis of their individual strengths and weaknesses. In short, it was hoped that the Pennsylvania Experiment would significantly alter the quality of life in dental school, which many educators and practitioners perceive as needing improvement.

Small clinical settings were also expected to allow students and faculty to place priority on the treatment of patients rather than on fulfilling requirements for students' graduation. Many faculty members and students refer to a "dental school mentality" in some schools, in which priority is given to checking off procedures rather than to treating patients. The experimental settings were designed to create a more professional environment.

Finally, perhaps the greatest educational innovation in the Pennsylvania Experiment was the implementation of the preceptor model of education. Unlike

THE PENNSYLVANIA EXPERIMENT

medical education, in which students learn by watching and then doing, students in dental schools rarely have the opportunity to observe faculty members in practice. Universities gather highly talented and respected clinicians on their faculties, yet students go through four years of dental school without ever witnessing them directly in practice. Excellent clinicians assume only supervisory roles in students' clinical education. Rather than demonstrating techniques directly, they teach students using slides and then supervise student activity in the clinic. The creators of the experiment believed this system was not only ineffective educationally but a patent waste of the talents and skills of dental school faculty members. In the new program, students received their clinical education with practicing master clinicians, observing and practicing with faculty members directly.

In summary, the Pennsylvania Experiment was designed to produce the dentist of the future in the most effective and efficient way possible, using faculty resources fully, and addressing current financial and fiscal problems—all within a humane, socially responsible environment. The synthesis of these diverse elements into one cohesive program did not happen rapidly or easily. To understand the origins of the Pennsylvania Experiment fully, it is necessary to go back ten years to the beginning of a new administration at the University of Pennsylvania School of Dental Medicine.

Notes

1. Richard S. MacKenzie, "The Role of Curriculum and Faculty Evaluation in Dental Education," *Journal of Dental Education* 45, no. 10 (1981): 678–82.
2. D. W. Cohen, P. Cormier, et al. "Predictions About the Future of Dental Education and Practice by Leaders in Dental Education: An Assessment of the Assumptions Underlying the Pennsylvania Experiment." Unpublished survey, 1980.
3. Charles Jerge et al., eds. *Group Practice and the Future of Dental Care.* Philadelphia: Lea and Febiger, 1974.
4. David W. Strevel, "Consumer Choice Between Dental Delivery Systems," *Journal of the American Dental Association* 104, no. 2 (February 1982): 157–63.
5. Committee on the Future of Dentistry, "Preliminary Strategic Plan," April 1983.
6. Frederick M. Parkins, "The Impact of Declining Resources on Dental Education," *Journal of Dental Education* 45, no. 10 (1981): 646–51.
7. Committee on the Future of Dentistry, "Preliminary Strategic Plan," p. 8.
8. American Association of Dental Schools, "Proceedings of the AADS Conference: General Practice Residency and Advanced General Dentistry Programs," *Journal of Dental Education* 47, no. 10 (1983).
9. Cohen, Cormier, et al., "Predictions About the Future," p. 5.
10. C. W. Douglass and J. M. Day, "Cost and Payment of Dental Services in the U.S.," *Journal of Dental Education* 43, no. 7 (1979): 330–46.
11. Morton Amsterdam, "The Future Role of the Generalist," Keynote Address, Yale University Conference on the Future of the Generalist, February 28, 1975.

12. Committee on the Future of Dentistry, "Preliminary Strategic Plan," p. 10.
13. I. L. Kerr, "The Changing Character of Dental Practice and Its Impact on Dental Education," *Journal of Dental Education* 45, no. 10 (1981): 638–43.
14. S. R. Dworkin, "Behavioral Studies in Dental Eduction: Past, Present and Future," *Journal of Dental Education* 45, no. 10 (1981): 692–98.

Background of the Experiment, Part I: 1972–1976, Early Efforts Toward Change

On July 1, 1972, a new administration assumed leadership of the University of Pennsylvania School of Dental Medicine, headed by Dean D. Walter Cohen. Because the school was suffering from chronic problems, the environment was opportune for the large-scale changes that were about to occur in its program and facilities.

By the early 1970s, the student population at Pennsylvania had become increasingly large: as of 1973, 316 students received their clinical education in a building that contained only 240 operatories. This trend showed no signs of reversing itself; federal capitation requirements stipulated yearly increases in the student body (based on the Carnegie Report of 1970, which had predicted future shortages of health personnel). The school's physical facilities were grossly inadequate; the main Evans Building was more than sixty years old and contained outdated equipment and antiquated, costly utility and heating systems. The other large facility at the school, the Levy Oral Health Sciences Building, opened in 1969, had reached its space limitation by 1972. Inadequate facilities often directly impeded innovation at the school; for example, Pennsylvania was unable to implement a program in four-handed sit-down dentistry, a style of delivery that was becoming widespread in dental education and practice, because of its limited physical resources.

Dental education at Penn was also characterized by many of the problems that were common throughout the nation's dental schools. As mentioned in Chapter 1, although the goal of predoctoral education is to produce a generalist, most schools compartmentalize their curricula into separate departments for each specialty area, creating a fragmented approach to dentistry. Fragmentation was also a problem in other areas of the curriculum: between the basic and clinical sciences and between preclinical and clinical learning. Further, although the professional environment had changed dramatically in the past ten to twenty years, most schools, including Penn, still did not prepare their students adequately for the realities of practice management, dental insurance, and other complex aspects of professional life they would inevitably face after graduation.

Nevertheless, many innovations in dental education were beginning to surface throughout the country's schools of dentistry. During the 1960s and 1970s
some exciting trends had begun in dental education. Courses in behavioral
principles of dental practice, the application of behavioral principles to the care
of patients, community dentistry, forensic dentistry and medicine, and practice management were now being offered at most U.S. dental schools. Innovations such as early and multiple tracking opportunities and some dissolution
of traditional departmental structures and interdepartmental barriers by teaching courses on an interdepartmental basis were challenging the much-
criticized "lock-step" approach to dental education, in which students follow
a routine path through dental school. Several successful innovative experiments had been conducted in dental education, featuring concepts such as the
self-paced curriculum and comprehensive treatment of patients. Competency-
based education and developmental approaches in teacher education had also
appeared. Indeed, dental education in 1972 was enjoying a climate of change
and innovation.

In the spring of 1972, in preparation for a $255 million capital fund drive for
the 1980s, the university sent members of its Development Commission to
the school to report on its status. The commission issued a report in January
1973, which stated, "The School of Dental Medicine has long had an excellent
national reputation. Its external reputation has declined somewhat in recent
years."[1] This report confirmed that the time had come for a serious examination of the overall programs and direction of the School of Dental Medicine.

Thus the new administration assumed leadership of a school in need of improvement during an era that offered many opportunities. Dean Cohen brought
a history of imagination and creativity in dental education to his new position.
Some clues to the nature of this innovative quality and to the changes that
would occur at Pennsylvania during the next decade can be found in examining
his acceptance remarks upon appointment as dean, December 15, 1971. He
stated:

> The Faculty of the School of Dental Medicine is currently asking the
> question, "What will the practice of dental medicine be in twenty years,
> and what should the educational program be to meet those needs?" I
> hope the faculty will be responsive and bold enough to break the con-
> stricting mold of traditional educational patterns and allow for the more
> flexible development of the potentials of the student. During the past
> two years, experimental procedures at the school have shown the possi-
> bilities for, and value of, multiple track curricula. . . . I look forward to
> greater cooperation with the University at large, to take advantage of the
> many resources that can help dental school graduates make more signif-
> icant contributions in oral health care. . . . In order to improve delivery
> of oral health care to the population at large and to make the best use of
> manpower, dental students, hygiene students, dental assistants, and lab-
> oratory technicians will be trained together at the undergraduate level

to work in teams. . . . *The dental school also hopes to establish an intramural practice facility which could become a Mayo Clinic of Dentistry for patients with difficult oral problems.* . . . The University of
Pennsylvania School of Dental Medicine looks forward to assuming an
international position of pre-eminence in dental education.[2]

All of these points were to influence dental education at Pennsylvania during the next ten years. Of particular significance, however, were his words
about a "Mayo Clinic of Dentistry." This remark reflected a long-standing vision that had begun twenty years earlier.

In the early 1950s, Morton Amsterdam, then at Temple University, and D.
Walter Cohen began collaborating to develop a form of dental treatment that
could be used for dentitions that had been mutilated by dental caries and advanced periodontal disease. Known as "periodontal prosthesis," this form of
dentistry drew upon years of study and research in general dentistry and in
specialty areas such as endodontics, prosthodontics, orthodontics, and oral
surgery, as well as periodontology, resulting in an integration of the specialties
into a field of "total dentistry." Cohen and Amsterdam presented course material in periodontal prosthesis at both Pennsylvania and Temple. The key feature of their teaching approach was the use of preceptorship, in which students
studied in their teachers' dental practices, witnessing them treating patients.
Graduate students in periodontology and periodontal prosthesis brought their
patients to Amsterdam's and Cohen's private practices, consulting with them,
using their laboratories, and observing advanced cases of treatment under the
skilled hands of the faculty-practitioner.

It was soon evident that the preceptorship method produced very promising
results. Many of the early preceptees went on to distinguished careers in research, practice, and education. Seeing the value of this educational approach,
Cohen and Amsterdam began to envision extending preceptorship on a larger
scale. They investigated properties near the dental school, hoping to relocate
their practices within easy access of the school. Increasing numbers of students participated as preceptees in their practices; exceptional predoctoral can-
didates as well as graduate students were soon studying there. Out of these
educational experiments grew the idea of a Mayo Clinic of Dentistry, perceived
as the counterpart of the Mayo Clinic of Medicine in which the finest clinicians in their respective fields work together in one facility, providing superior
care to patients from around the world. The Mayo Clinic of Dentistry would
be affiliated with the School of Dental Medicine, so that students as well as
patients could benefit from a wealth of knowledge and skill. This idea was still
very alive in both Dr. Cohen's and Dr. Amsterdam's minds in 1972. Furthermore, several faculty members at Pennsylvania now shared this dream, having
been reared in the Periodontal Prosthesis Program.

In 1971 the search committee for a new dean had issued a curriculum report
aimed at educating the dentist of the future, who was defined as "a scholar; a

deliverer of health services to the community, cognizant of the known varied systems for health service delivery, and educated in the processes of defining the health needs of his/her community; a team leader, delegating appropriate tasks to auxiliaries; organizing, coordinating and leading the team, assuming primary responsibilities for general patient evaluation, diagnosis and treatment planning; and a member of the professional health team."[3] The committee proposed several alternatives to the traditional program of clinical education at Penn, one of which included a network of dental team units in which faculty members would have responsibility for the treatment of patients.

Thus the administration assumed leadership of a school in need of basic improvements during an era conducive to change and innovation. This new administration was committed to educating dentists prepared to meet the demands of the future and was endowed with its own particular dream about the future of dental education. The story of the Pennsylvania Experiment is one of the interweaving of that dream with the creative ideas and dreams of the faculty and with existing trends in dental education and in society, resulting in a new form of education at the School of Dental Medicine.

Early Improvements at the School of Dental Medicine

Beginning in 1972, efforts were made to address some of the chronic problems at Penn. In 1972, the firm of Hay Associates was engaged to recommend organizational and managerial improvements at the school. The consultants interviewed faculty and students and on the basis of their extensive survey concluded that the school had great potential, stating that it was "a professional school strongly anchored in the important history of dental care . . . that saw clearly the outlines of the future of dental medicine and that was already working to define its contributions at the frontier of health care."[4] The report made some major recommendations, including the establishment of two top administrative positions to assist the dean, centralization of clinic operations, and improvement in the student-faculty ratio. During the first year of the administration's tenure, the school was reorganized along these principles.

The problem of inadequate facilities was also addressed immediately; as early as 1972, a new eight-story facility was proposed. While these plans were under discussion, improvements and additions to the existing facilities were being made. In September 1972 the Myers Clinic, designed to educate graduate students in periodontal prosthesis, was dedicated, thereby consolidating the school's commitment to and preeminence in this field of total dentistry. The four-chair Morton Crossman Comprehensive Oral Health Clinic was dedicated in the spring of 1973 to train predoctoral and postgraduate students in comprehensive treatment procedures. In July 1976 the Mary and George Coleman Pediatric Center, consisting of twenty-five operatories as well as preventive and interceptive orthodontic facilities, was dedicated. The clinic used the team approach in the treatment of children and adolescents. An expanded undergraduate periodontal surgery facility (the Robinson Clinic), a new audiovisual learning laboratory, and the Abram Cohen Preventive Health Education Center were among the new facilities constructed, and the new preclinical teaching laboratory, the Alumni and Admissions Office, and office spaces for additional faculty were renovated.

Changes in the academic arena also moved the dental school toward increased flexibility and a program for educating the dentist of the future. Multiple-track programs (including combined D.M.D./Ph.D., D.M.D./M.B.A., and D.M.D./M.D. programs) were established. A Department of Dental Care Systems was added to the school to define the requirements of a viable dental care delivery system for the future and to teach students about issues such as practice organization and financing, manpower requirements, patient care quality assessment, and information systems to monitor performance. Courses given by this department would help prepare students for careers in an increasingly complex dental practice environment. Other academic changes included consolidation of the departments of Pharmacology and Physiology and combining the departments of Pedodontics and Orthodontics to form a Department of Pediatric Dentistry, thereby helping to reduce fragmentation.

In 1974–75, an important change occurred in the academic structure of the school, which was to lead to even greater innovations in the future. An experimental group practice in general dentistry for the teaching of undergraduate clinical dentistry was implemented on the main clinic floor. Students were assigned to a specific group of faculty members who worked consistently with them throughout their clinical years. This innovation was a marked departure from the organization of the traditional clinic, in which students and faculty are randomly assigned to a bay of chairs each semester. The group practice also featured an improved student-faculty ratio and fewer rotations outside of the main clinic, resulting in provision of more comprehensive care in one setting. Under the leadership of Drs. Daniel Casullo and Francis Matarazzo, two graduates of the Periodontal Prosthesis Graduate Program, the program was highly successful in its second year. After three years, the entire main clinic was converted to a series of group practices in response to the demand of students, who viewed the new program as highly desirable.

Long-Range Planning (1974–1976)

In January 1974, an event occurred that was to synthesize many of these efforts toward change, ultimately resulting in a new form of dental education at Penn-

sylvania. On January 8, the trustees of the University of Pennsylvania committed themselves to a major fund-raising drive and mandated formation of a
long-range planning committee to develop a blueprint for the future of the
major health schools of the university.

In response to this request, the dental school formed a Long Range Planning
Committee composed of key faculty members (see Appendix I). The committee developed a preliminary plan identifying two major goals for the school: an
improvement in the student-faculty ratio and the provision of physical facilities of clinical instruction conducive with current and projected oral health
care delivery systems. The construction of an eight-story building to house
additional clinical as well as teaching and research facilities was proposed, in
addition to renovations to the Evans Building. The committee viewed gradual
increase in the number of fully affiliated faculty members as necessary to improve the student-faculty ratio. On May 24, 1974, the report of the Long Range
Planning Committee was submitted to Dr. Thomas Langfitt, vice-president for
health affairs. Dr. Langfitt gave the plans preliminary approval, and the committee continued to meet to develop a more comprehensive program based on
these recommendations.

The committee soon recognized this task as an opportunity for serious self-
study and long-range planning. Rather than creating hypothetical plans, the
school chose to develop a well-defined course of action for the future. The
efforts of the committee were extended in 1975. A comprehensive plan for the
future of the School of Dental Medicine, based on existing trends in society
and in the dental health profession, would be developed, using a two-pronged
approach. The Task Force on the Academic Future of the School of Dental
Medicine (see Appendix II) was formed to propose future academic programs,
and the Perreault Health Planning Agency of Washington, D.C., was engaged
to study and propose options for future facilities at the school. Large-scale
planning for the comprehensive restructuring of the school was under way.

TASK FORCE ON FUTURE ACADEMIC PROGRAMS
OF THE SCHOOL OF DENTAL MEDICINE

The task force was charged by the dean with the mission of developing future
academic programs at the School of Dental Medicine "for the remaining quarter of this century (1975–2000)." His letter to the task force stated:

> Traditionally, institutions devoted to dental education have not been sig-
> nificantly sensitive to the changing conditions of the external environ-
> ment—conditions which should legitimately influence an institution's
> objectives in education, research and service. The current period is one
> of more rapid change in health care than any similar time in history. . . .
> The time has come for a coordinated group to look intensively and ana-
> lytically into the strengths and weaknesses of the School's various aca-

demic programs, and to utilize this information in helping to plan the mission of the School of Dental Medicine for the remainder of this millenium. . . . Hopefully, we will structure an institution that does not yet exist in this country and which, if successful, will become the model for others to follow."[5]

Figure 2-1. Historical Development of the Pennsylvania Experiment, Part I: 1974–1976

July 1974	University requested all health schools to form a long-range planning committee to develop a "blueprint for the future" as part of its $255 million capital drive.
May 1975	Long Range Planning Committee of the School of Dental Medicine presented a preliminary report to the university, calling for a new facility and an improvement in the student-faculty ratio.
September 1975	School of Dental Medicine extended its planning efforts, using a twofold approach:
	—Task Force on the Academic Future of the School of Dental Medicine formed to develop a blueprint for the academic future of the school.
	—Perreault Health Planning Agency engaged to develop facilities plans for the future of the school.
October 1975	Task Force on the Academic Future of the School disbanded because of conflict with the university over the issue of reducing class size.
June 1976	Perreault Report on facilities improvements at the school submitted, recommending several alternatives, including an east courtyard in-fill and a new eight-story facility.
June 1976	Faculty Senate of the School of Dental Medicine approved the Perreault Report "in principle" but requested additional plans for the future of the academic program at the School of Dental Medicine.

The task force was chaired by Dr. Charles Jerge, whose career path had great impact on its direction. Dr. Jerge had been trained at Pennsylvania as a preceptee in periodontal prosthesis, while pursuing his Ph.D. in neurophysiology. He had gone on to become dean of the dental school at the University of Connecticut before returning to Penn to chair the newly formed Department of Dental Care Systems. Well known for his work on alternative modes of delivery in health care, Dr. Jerge brought an innovative, forward-looking approach to the committee. The task force was composed of sixteen other faculty members and administrators.

After convening on September 12, 1975, the task force met for one month, studying a variety of materials concerning trends and issues in health care delivery. Basic questions relating to the academic future of the school were discussed. The committee asked: What type of dentist will be required for the future? What is the optimal size of each of the desired programs in dental education (predoctoral, graduate, and auxiliary) to achieve quality and balance? What is the optimal setting for each of these programs? After several meetings and discussions, the committee developed four alternative programs based on four basic premises about the future of dentistry. These premises formed the foundation of the committee's plans and of plans that were developed by succeeding planning committees. By basing its plan on this foundation, the school would develop a program that would be responsive to future societal trends and needs.

The four basic premises were as follows: (1) Group practice and other forms of institutionalized health care will gradually replace solo practice; (2) Dental care will gradually merge into comprehensive primary care organizations, and team health care will replace referral of patients among isolated practitioners; (3) Four factors—the growth of group practice, the integration of dental care into comprehensive health organizations, the expanded role of auxiliaries in dental care, and financing mechanisms to control costs—will create conditions that will lessen the need for dental specialists and heighten the need for well-trained general dentists; (4) Therefore, at least 80 percent of graduates of D.M.D. and advanced training programs should be general dentists with more clinical training than current dental graduates receive. They should be well prepared to work in an interdisciplinary health care team, in a dental care team (dentists and auxiliaries), and in a group practice setting. Anyone so prepared can adapt to solo practice if desired; the converse is not so easy.

A reduction in class size was also central to the committee's discussions. Earlier attempts to improve the student-faculty ratio had focused on increasing the number of faculty members. By 1975 it had become clear that the school was overcrowded and that a reduction in class size was a more logical solution. Further, the committee members, as well as many dental educators, were beginning to question the underlying assumption of federal capitation requirements that a health manpower shortage was imminent. The role of the general dentist seemed to be changing toward providing a greater scope of services traditionally assigned to the specialist, which meant that there was no longer a need to produce large numbers of dental professionals. Many members of the committee had begun to question the wisdom of continuing to receive capitation funds because this system imposed a situation of overcrowding and poor educational conditions on the school. In addition, federal funding from capitation had been decreasing steadily since 1973. In that year, funding was at a 62 percent level of regional funding; in 1975, funding was at a 47.5 percent level.

On September 30, 1975, Vice-President for Health Affairs Thomas Langfitt met with the task force and informed them that they must not include reduction in class size in future discussions. The university believed that its health schools should continue to meet federal health manpower requirements so that federal funds would not be jeopardized.

Feeling strongly that a reduction in class size was essential, the committee unanimously voted to dissolve following the university's ultimatum. Long-range planning for the academic future of the school had temporarily come to a halt.

PERREAULT HEALTH PLANNING AGENCY

The Perreault Health Planning Agency was retained in the fall of 1975 to accomplish the second half of the planning process: developing plans to meet the school's needs for facilities. The agency interviewed faculty, students, and administrators to identify the needs and issues upon which any long-range plan for the facilities of the school should be based. The report identified nine major needs; many of them were in harmony with the premises developed by the Task Force on the Academic Future of the School. Five proposals were then made for improving the facilities at the school, which the Perreault group confirmed were badly in need of renovation or replacement. These proposals ranged from renovating existing facilities to constructing an in-fill to the east courtyard of the school.

On June 9, 1976, the dean sent a letter to the Faculty Senate, requesting its attendance at an important meeting on June 23, at which the recommendations of the Perreault Agency would be presented for its consideration. The dean's letter began as follows:

> I am thoroughly convinced that we have made some very good decisions in the past few years and by means of new programs, individuals and research activities, we have strengthened the School of Dental Medicine. However, we must realize that this is not nearly enough when one attempts to assay the potential of this school as an integral part of one of the outstanding institutions of higher learning in the history of the United States . . . we as a faculty can and must advance our school to a position of preeminence in dental education by fully realizing the potential that exists within the student body, staff and faculty. . . . Planning for change means a great deal of effort, and I am going to ask you to deliberate more about where the University of Pennsylvania School of Dental Medicine can and will be in the remaining quarter of this century than you have ever had to do in the past.[6]

The following key points were outlined as areas of future change in dental education at Penn: developing an oral biology track to bring together clinicians and basic scientists and enhance the teaching program; familiarizing dental students with the concept of the oral health team and use of expanded-function dental auxiliaries; exposing students to the most modern methods of health care delivery; familiarizing students with the realities of practice management in a group or solo environment; and allowing students to learn directly from a preceptorship mode of education. The letter emphasized this last point:

What I perceive to be our greatest deficiency is our entire system of training clinicians. Except for our general practice group, the average student does not observe the master clinicians on our faculty treating patients. Our clinical teachers at the predoctoral level are in the main individuals who check procedures but do not demonstrate for the student. To my way of thinking, it is completely absurd to assemble the most distinguished clinical faculty and have the students only observe their clinical skills by showing a carousel tray of slides. It is time that we completely revamp the entire process of the making of a dentist. The student has to be placed into an environment that is modern in every sense of the word, and see this delivery system from his/her first year at the school. He/she should hold the retractors and pass instruments for our faculty so that the master clinician can truly be a role model. Our students should also be able to step aside and see the entire dental team in action. All of our new clinical faculty should understand that their teaching role is given to encompass demonstrations and they should be prepared to switch positions at the chair and coach the student through a procedure while they are assisting the novice. This approach is going to require that we establish a facility on the campus that will enable our faculty to engage in clinical practice wherein undergraduates as well as postgraduate students will rotate in a fashion similar to that of the hospital and extramural assignments that we have required of each of our graduates during the past four years. This task is going to be a mammoth one since we are dealing with more than 300 predoctoral students in their clinical years. However, I remain firmly convinced that when we accomplish this it will be our greatest contribution to dentistry and will result in a renaissance for dental education at the School. I am also convinced that we will be able to pass on to our followers a system of education that is sound from an academic and fiscal basis.[7]

On June 23, 1976, the Faculty Senate met to consider the recommendations of the Perreault Report and the principles it embodied. The senate concluded that it approved of the Perreault Report "in principle." It also stated, however, that in order to make specific decisions about constructing a new facility or renovating the existing one, it needed more specific information about the corresponding academic plan that was to be implemented.

In response, in July 1976, a Long Range Planning Committee was formed to develop an academic plan for the future of the School of Dental Medicine. Once again, a group of faculty members and administrators sat down to develop a blueprint for the future of education at the school.

Notes

1. University Development Commission, "Pennsylvania, One University," *Almanac* 19, no. 30 (January 1973).

2. D. W. Cohen, "Acceptance Remarks," December 15, 1971 (unpublished).
3. Educational Policy Subcommittee, "Report of the Educational Policy Subcommittee," September 8, 1971.
4. Hay Associates, "Organization and Management Processes Study: University of Pennsylvania School of Dental Medicine," June 1972, p. 1.
5. D. W. Cohen, "Charge to the Task Force on the Future of Academic Programs at the School of Dental Medicine, for the Remaining Quarter of this Century (1975–2000)," September 3, 1975.
6. D. W. Cohen, Letter to the Faculty Senate, June 9, 1976.
7. Ibid.

3

Background of the Experiment, Part II: 1976– 1978: The Pennsylvania Experiment Is Born

During the summer of 1976, the Long Range Planning Committee began meeting to develop an academic program based on the principles embodied in the Perreault Report. Composed of many of the members of the disbanded Task Force on the Future of Academic Programs, the committee also included Maurice Perreault of the Perreault Health Planning Agency and Dale Wade of the university's Department of Facilities Development, along with several other new members (see Appendix III). The discussions of the Long Range Planning Committee centered around many of the issues that had been discussed by the task force the previous fall.

Several new developments on the national level supported the direction of the committee. In October 1976 the Carnegie Commission on Higher Education reversed its previous position, now suggesting that an undersupply of health professionals was no longer a concern. Further, in the fall 1976, the U.S. General Accounting Office (GAO) issued a report warning of a possible oversupply of physicians and dentists. The general national concern had shifted from one of avoiding an undersupply toward preventing an oversupply of health professionals. In addition, capitation funding to dental schools had continued to decline. No longer was the possible cessation of federal funding because of a reduction in class size a major issue; funds were gradually being reduced anyway. These factors strengthened the committee's stand on a reduced class size, removing a major barrier to implementing this aspect of the school's long-range plans.

On January 12, 1977, the Long Range Planning Committee submitted a report to the Faculty Senate, including an explication of the current perceived problems within health care delivery and dental education and proposed solutions. The report called for a reorientation toward the education of a highly competent dental generalist prepared to function in a group setting. It went on to delineate the specific tasks that this "expert dentist" would perform.

With auxiliaries assuming responsibility for basic preventive and restorative care, the expert dentist would be responsible for functional disorders of the stomatognathic system, advanced periodontal disease, replacement of missing

23

teeth, trauma affecting the dentition and adjacent soft tissues, and oral lesions other than malignancies and those requiring complex surgical interventions. Having been trained to assume some of the skills of the current dental specialist, the expert dentist would have one or more areas of particular expertise; among these would be advanced restorative procedures (fixed and removable prosthesis), periodontics, endodontics, basic orthodontics, and basic oral surgery. He/she would also be trained in multiple clinical environments, including the hospital, and "should develop a broad perspective on patient needs, and above all must develop a high level of clinical competence in the relevant areas of general dental practice."[1] Advanced aspects of oral surgery such as maxillo-facial reconstruction and the management of severe trauma would be performed by hospital-based specialists, and prosthodontics would continue to be an area of expertise for some general dentists, although it was hoped that prosthetics would gradually decline in the future as preventive dental technologies had an effect on the general level of oral health of the population.

Thirteen proposals were then made for a new curriculum, including a smaller class size, improved faculty-student ratios, a preceptor mode of clinical education, and several other key points. The issue of the financial feasibility of the new program was also addressed in this report. The major fiscal question was the impact that a reduction in class size would have on the economics of the school. The report concluded that the plan was financially feasible but predicted that reduction of numbers of students would require a tuition increase. This increase could be moderated by additional income from the proposed faculty practices, from the use of clinical faculty members who would offset part or all of their costs by generating income in one of the school's faculty practices, and from a substantial decrease in indirect cost charges for utilities and housekeeping once the class size had been reduced and subsequent renovation of the main (Evans) building had been accomplished.

The report, submitted on January 12, 1977, was accepted with some minor recommendations for change; on March 9, 1977, a revised presentation was accepted fully by the Faculty Senate. After more than four years of discussions and proposals, the School of Dental Medicine had received approval from its faculty for a comprehensive plan for the future of its educational programs. These recommendations were to become the outline for the Pennsylvania Experiment. Because of their significance to the experiment, they are included here in full.

Report of the Long Range Planning Committee

THE EDUCATIONAL MISSION OF THE SCHOOL OF DENTAL MEDICINE (1979)

The educational mission of the School of Dental Medicine is to prepare the types of health professionals who will most adequately meet the future requirements of our society. The University of Pennsylvania is committed to achieving the maximum oral "fitness" for the greatest number of citizens, children and adults through prevention, treatment, and research. Successful dental practice arrangements in the future will involve highly competent generalists, dental specialists, and dental auxiliary therapists, functioning in complementary roles. The principal thrust of the educational effort of the school will be directed toward training highly competent generalists with programs for dental specialists and dental auxiliary training. University practice models for faculty and students will be adapted to meet the needs of the educational programs of the school, with the view of creating practice settings most ideal for the training of future practitioners.

The following recommendations are intended to implement this commitment of the School of Dental Medicine.

Recommendation 1:   That the class be reduced to eighty students (80) beginning with the class entering in the fall of 1979.

The inadequacy of the faculty/student ratio (1:12) caused by the current class size makes achievement of the educational objectives extremely difficult if not impossible. The overcrowding of the facility due to the current class size makes preclinical and clinical programs inefficient and the teaching of multi-handed, sit-down dentistry in a modern practice setting unachievable for the majority of the students.

Recommendation 2:   That the School of Dental Medicine begin a new curriculum in the Fall of 1979 which will include a fifth year family practice residency program.

At the end of the Fourth Year the DMD degree will be awarded. The students at the end of the fourth year will have a broadened background in the basic sciences and more and better quality clinical training than the current graduates. The fifth year residency, which is hospital and school based, is planned for students who will be designated as Family Practice Generalists. This program will not be compulsory. There will be a stipend, waiver of tuition, and virtually a full commitment to dental practice and clinical services so that the generalist is highly competent in several specialties.

Transfer to specialty training programs at the end of the fourth year will also be possible.

Recommendation 3:   That the preceptorship model of clinic instruction be adopted as the principal method of clinical instruction and that clinic based (as exemplified by the current student General Group Practice) and faculty group practice based preceptorship teams will constitute the normative clinical experiences for the student.

The Committee recommends that clinical instruction be organized around preceptorship teams in Family Practice Groups which in the beginning will be clinic-based and much like the current student General Group Practice. The Family Practice will treat both children and adults. The preceptors are to participate within the teams and are to be accountable for the patient care provided. As the intramural, full-time clinical faculty practice(s) grow, students will gradually be transferred to the faculty practice(s), which may be part of a network of practices located at sites in addition to 40th and Spruce Streets.

Preceptorship teams will include dental auxiliaries, dental hygiene students, first, second, third, and fourth year dental students and Family Practice Residents. Dental students in years 1 and 2 will spend ½ to 1 day per week in a preceptorship team. Third and fourth year students will spend most of their time in a preceptorship team but will have oral biology courses, elective course and research opportunities and extramural (including hospital) clinical rotations. The residents in the Family Group Practice will rotate between preceptorship teams and hospital practice.

Recommendation 4:   That a system of faculty group practices, under the aegis of the University and staffed by full time clinical faculty be instituted, wherein the clinical instruction of the future will take place; all of the current clinic patients would ultimately become patients of the faculty group practices and a significant portion of the clinic income would be derived from the practices.

This recommendation is viewed as imperative because the phasing out of clinic-type operations is occurring and will accelerate as dental insurance and other third party programs grow. The relationship of faculty practice to preceptorship education is also of central importance. In the long run, the strength of preceptorship education will rest on the strength and economic viability of a faculty practice system.

Recommendation 5:   That the preclinical technique course be revised to stress the learning of those basic skills which students will be called upon to apply in the immediate future and to relate the technique course in time to the developing clinical experiences of the student.

Training shall be closer to practice situations and techniques. Observation in the clinic of techniques will be correlated with techniques being studied in the laboratory and with rapid transition into clinical experience.

Recommendation 6:   That the curriculum of the first four years be a balanced experience to broaden the background of the generalist (and reduce the emphasis on the specialties as separate entities).

The following elements are to be included:

• Basic Sciences

Courses should be examined to keep to a minimum redundancy with previous student courses and among basic science courses.

• Interdisciplinary Oral Biology Courses throughout the entire program

Rather than attempt to provide a complete program of Oral Biology courses which would conflict with many of the basic science programs, selected topics in Oral Biology will be the focus. This will allow for the development of those areas of dental science which have significant content and which are multidisciplinary in nature. Oral Biology will thus be limited to selected topics rather than representing a course of instruction. This arrangement will permit the most pertinent and well developed areas of oral science to be coordinated with clinical components.

• Behavioral and Social Sciences, Patient Management Core Sequence

- Practice Organization and Management, Dental Auxiliary Utilization, Training in Experimental Auxiliary Management, and a Health Care Issues and Systems Core Sequence

  These two "core" course series are important in preparing the student to deal successfully with the individual patient, the challenges of practice organization and operation and the changing dimensions of health services delivery.
- Preparation for the Clinic

  Revised Preclinical Technique Course combined with integrated and correlated clinical observation and participation will be implemented.
- Clinic Experience

  It is planned that the first year students will have about 10–15% of their time in the clinic as observers and as members of the teams. By the fourth year, approximately 75% of student time will be in the clinics.
- Elective Opportunities in Behavioral and Social Sciences, in the Clinic Specialties, in Clinical and Basic Science Research, and in other courses of the University shall be included.

  Adequate time, but no less than 15% in each of the first four years, is to be available for electives within the School and/or the University.

Recommendation 7: That the academic calendar of the School of Dental Medicine be made to conform to the undergraduate calendar of the University, and that the calendar should furthermore be arranged so that each semester is subdivided into two parts for mini-courses, particularly electives.

The intent is to foster courses of fewer than sixteen weeks' duration. The academic year would consist of five instructional periods, two each during the fall and spring semesters, and one during a summer session. Many of the required courses and all of the elective courses would be programmed into an eight-week format and offered with a frequency such that students on extramural rotations would be able to select from a complete list of course offerings. Extramural student rotations would conform to the same calendar as the formal course offerings.

In addition, more flexibility in taking courses outside of the School of Dental Medicine will be possible, and conforming to the undergraduate calendar will encourage a greater overall sharing of academic experiences within the University.

Recommendation 8: That the training of dental specialists be continued, with a cautious eye on the changing character of dental practice and that the consequent need to alter or phase out specific specialty training programs as appropriate action for the future be considered.

The School of Dental Medicine has established its reputation in large part on the excellence of its specialty training programs. Requirements for specialists are changing, however, and some regions of the country are already saturated with oral surgeons, endodontists, periodontists, and orthodontists. The School should continue cautiously its current programs, should continue to experiment with combining specialty programs and should establish a leadership role in defining the types and roles of specialists required for the future. The specialists (postdoctoral students and faculty) will provide care at the specialty level for patients in the Family Practice Group.

Recommendation 9:   That dental auxiliary education in the School be integrated with the clinical education of the dental students, that a comprehensive plan be developed for dental hygiene education involving basic preparation and possible baccalaureate and master's degree level programs and that a study be made of the feasibility of increasing the number of dental auxiliary students prepared with the dental students for efficient team practice.

An important focus of this Long Range Plan relates to the changing requirements of dental practice and the increasing importance of defining the optimum role of dental auxiliary personnel in dental care. The reduction in class size of dental students, and the adoption of team teaching and preceptorship instruction afford an excellent opportunity for innovation in dental auxiliary education.

Recommendation 10:   That mechanisms be implemented concurrently with the new programs to ensure (a) achievement of the recommendations, (b) adjustments where objectives are not achieved, (c) instructional quality, (d) student performance evaluation, and (e) quality of patient care.

In any program as far reaching as herein proposed, built-in mechanisms must be included in the planning to judge the success or failure of the various components of the program. Mechanisms for adjustments and mid-course corrections must also be built-in.

The potential success of the new clinical program has been defined in terms of the new delivery systems, which are dependent on the expertise of clinicians in patient care. The Long Range Planning Committee is cognizant of the fact that there might not be a direct correlation between distinguished teaching and clinical or research competence and recommends that a mechanism to monitor teaching and program effectiveness as measured by student competency in this new modality be implemented concurrent with the implementation of the new curriculum. Such a system will ensure that the objectives of the new program are maintained and enhanced.

Recommendation 11:   That, with the reduction in the number of students, a major renovation of the Evans Building plus the necessity of an east court in-fill and/or a faculty practice facility will serve the needs of the School if the above recommendations are approved.

Approved by

Faculty Senate of the
University of Pennsylvania
School of Dental Medicine[2]

March 9, 1977

Figure 3-1. Historical Development of the Pennsylvania Experiment, Part II: 1976–1978

July 1976	Second Long Range Planning Committee formed in response to Faculty Senate's request for an academic plan for the future of the school.
October 1976	Carnegie Commission reversed its previous warnings of an undersupply of health professionals, now predicting the opposite problem.
March 1977	Eleven recommendations of the Long Range Planning Committee for the school's future approved by Faculty Senate; School of Dental Medicine began planning a new program based on the Long Range Plan.
January 1978	School of Dental Medicine presented its Long Range Plan to Board of Trustees, University of Pennsylvania, and received an enthusiastic response.
May 1978	Educational Policy Committee of the university recommended that the school conduct a pilot study of the principles embodied in the Long Range Plan.
September 1978	School of Dental Medicine submitted a proposal to Pew Memorial Trust of the Glenmede Trust Company for a pilot study to test the Long Range Plan.
November 1978	Grant of $1 million awarded to School of Dental Medicine for a pilot study, to be known as the Pennsylvania Experiment.

Designing the New Program

After the Faculty Senate accepted its eleven recommendations, the Long Range Planning Committee began designing a comprehensive program that would incorporate the many changes prescribed. In September 1977, Dr. Stephen Wotman, then on sabbatical from his position as assistant dean for administration and planning at Columbia University's School of Dental and Oral Surgery, was asked to aid in the development of this new program.

THE PRACTICE HOUSE

The task of the Long Range Planning Committee was complicated because there were no precedents in dental education for some of the key components of the new program. No previous model existed, for example, of the faculty-based practice/educational unit. It was important that the program provide opportunities for a stable, controllable, and effective clinical teaching environment in which the affective aspects of dental education could be stressed. Therefore, a model had to be created from the ideas and knowledge of the committee and from the experience of institutions that had addressed similar issues. The device chosen was the collegiate structure of the English university, which had been adapted and modified for the University of California at Santa Cruz.[3] This model had not been used in professional education but seemed appropriate for the requirements of the Long Range Plan. The Santa Cruz planning documents describe the collegiate structure as follows:

> The most conspicuous feature of the Santa Cruz design was its collegiate structure. The campus would grow each year by adding a small, self-contained college. By 1970–71 there would be five colleges, each with from 550 to 700 students, that would share the common goals of providing quality undergraduate teaching and close relationships among students and faculty. The design was such that each college, distinctive in its own right, had an intellectual "center of gravity" which stemmed from the interests and activities of its members . . . by design, the collegiate structure permitted faculty to shape and to influence their own environment. It facilitated interdisciplinary teaching and research by bringing together faculty members from various disciplines. It was structured to create a feeling of belonging and intimacy through the small college without forfeiting the wide variety of subjects, the excellence of facilities, and the search for new knowledge that are part of a great university.[4]

The description was highly appropriate for the preceptor model in that it emphasized smallness and close contact between student and faculty members, who would interact together in a collegial relationship. It was also in keeping with the goals of the committee members to reduce the dehumanizing aspects of dental education.

To adapt the Santa Cruz model to the long-range plans of the School of Dental Medicine, the idea of a "practice house" was conceived. The practice house would be a faculty group practice, augmented by students from all classes, dental auxiliary students, and dental residents. It would be both an educational and a service institution, teaching dental skills firsthand within the small and real-life environment of the group practice. This practice would consist of several generalists and a few rotating specialists. It would serve a specific community and have a patient population of mixed economic background. Both fee-for-service and per capita payment arrangements would be used. The practice would be responsible for all services provided by an extended primary care dental organization and would assume either a referral, managerial, or partnership role with other health care components serving the same population. Students would participate in care depending upon their achievement level in a criterion-based curriculum. Practice house committees would deal with a variety of issues ranging from quality assurance to community action for preventive health. Students would be assigned to one practice house for their four years of clinical training, providing an opportunity for a collegial relationship between professor and student to mature.

The practice house would be financially supported through practice revenue (for services provided or through per capita contracts) and educational revenue (tuition) for the time students spent in it. Dental residents would have both teaching and service responsibilities.

The practice house was also seen as an opportune environment for explicit instruction in the behavioral sciences because it provided built-in role models for students. The organizational structure seemed to be ideal for the fulfillment of the recommendations of the Long Range Planning Committee.

FEASIBILITY STUDY

Dr. Wotman prepared a feasibility study of the new program based on the practice house model. Two basic types of practice houses were described: Model A would be a transitional unit patterned closely after the current group practice model that had been implemented on the main clinic floor. It would be a small clinical environment, emphasizing comprehensive care provided by residents and students under the close supervision and occasional participation of faculty. Model B would be a prototype of the generalist-oriented group practice of the future and would be staffed by faculty providers/teachers functioning as "master clinician" role models. The presence of full-time generalists would be complemented by full- or part-time specialists.

The feasibility study contained a theoretical model of the program, projecting staffing, costs, and revenue. Several elements of the plan were identified as being critical to its success. Among these were the formation of the Model B practice and its ability to produce revenue; the ability of the current faculty to carry out comprehensive care teaching in both the Models A and B practices; and the ability of the school to attract sufficient patients required by the addition of residents and practicing faculty to the school environment. The study also noted that it was essential that these decentralized educational units offer an education at least comparable to that of a traditional dental school. The success of the experiment would rest on the ability of a private practice to provide educational instruction without compromising patient care. All of these issues were cited as requiring further investigation if the Long Range Plan was to be academically and fiscally viable for the future of the school.[5]

UNIVERSITY RESPONSE

On January 12, 1978, the School of Dental Medicine presented its Long Range Plan for approval by the Board of Trustees of the University of Pennsylvania, chaired by Donald Regan. On January 18, University President Martin Meyerson submitted a letter to Dean Cohen, informing him of the trustees' response: "I was so pleased at your presentation of the Dental School's proposed new curriculum to the Trustees last Thursday. Everyone is captured by the boldness of the program you and your colleagues have devised."[6]

The letter went on to express the trustees' concerns about the fiscal viability of a drastic reduction in class size. Could the school balance its budget with such a large cutback in tuition dollars? Several board members suggested that a pilot study of the new plan on a small scale would be helpful for evaluating financial viability before a large-scale change in the curriculum was implemented.

Following this meeting, the plan was submitted to the University Senate's Educational Planning Committee (EPC) for its review. In May 1978, the committee expressed its support for the concepts embodied in the proposal but raised questions about the potential financial and academic consequences of the major changes that were recommended. Would the school have an adequate financial base when the class size was cut? Would the Model B practice generate enough revenue to be financially self-sustaining; that is, could a private practice sustain the presence of students and still maintain fiscal viability? What contingencies had been made for the immediate future of the school in light of the anticipated loss of federal capitation funds? The EPC felt that all of these questions must be answered before any large-scale changes were implemented at the school.

A PILOT STUDY

Accordingly, the Long Range Planning Committee began to investigate funding opportunities for a pilot study while it continued to meet to address the major issues of the new program.

Clinical-Educator Track

One such issue was the development of a proposal for a clinical educator career track as an alternative to the traditional tenure track. The new program centered around the acquisition of a faculty member who would both teach and practice and who therefore would have limited time to devote to research. To provide a secure career path for this faculty member, an alternative to the tenure track was necessary. Clinical practitioners within the university often faced tremendous difficulty in establishing careers; the tenure requirements of the university emphasized teaching and research and gave little recognition to service as a criterion for appointment and promotion. Young clinicians often recognized that in all likelihood they would be forced to relocate their careers at the time a tenure decision was made. Recognizing this situation, the School of Medicine had established a nontenure career track for its full-time clinical faculty, so that young physicians could concentrate on teaching and clinical practice if they chose. A clinical educator track was perceived as an important element in making the Model B faculty-based practice an attractive environment for clinician-educators.

Marketing Study

In May 1978, a marketing study of the West Philadelphia community was completed by the American Health and Management Consulting Corporation (AHMAC), directed by Dr. John Amsterdam, formerly a full-time faculty member at the School of Dental Medicine, to assess the market for a new Model B practice. The study analyzed the demography, the sources of financing dental care, and the supply and demand for dental service in West Philadelphia. Alternative marketing strategies for the Model B practice in West Philadelphia were also explored.

The analysis of the West Philadelphia market indicated that a substantial patient base existed in the residential and working populations and that at the time of the report there was a relative shortage of dental providers in the area. In addition, the School of Dental Medicine's proximity to and affiliations with the universities and hospitals that made up the university community provided a significant marketing advantage for gaining access to these student and employee groups. The AHMAC study projected that the patient market could support between eighteen and thirty full-time-equivalent (FTE) practitioners within the first three to five years of operation. The school had received a "go-ahead" in this important area, which was vital to the potential success of a Model B practice.[7]

Other Developments

Several subcommittees prepared and submitted reports on various aspects of the experiment. A preliminary curriculum guide for the new program, a fiscal study of the new Model B practice, and a study of the public relations needs of the practice were all prepared.

By May, the University Facilities Office had identified a potential site for the Model B faculty practice, conveniently located in a shopping center near the School of Dental Medicine complex. By September 1978, a study of the physical requirements of the new Model B facility had been completed, including a projected schedule of construction and a projected budget. The site was rented in December 1978.

Grant Proposal

In September 1978, a proposal was submitted to the Pew Memorial Trust of the Glenmede Trust Company for the funding of the pilot study to test the underlying concepts of the Long Range Plan. The proposal posed the following six issues as topics which the study would address: (1) assessing whether the new teaching program is more effective than existing traditional programs in producing competent students; (2) determining whether increased professional competence is accompanied by advanced technical skills; (3) judging whether the program's environment encourages students to orient themselves toward total and comprehensive patient care; (4) weighing how these new educational programs can be supported adequately by patient care revenues, an acceptable tuition, and realistic levels of other support with a reduced class size; (5) establishing whether the Long Range Plan's educational innovations are truly compatible with the University of Pennsylvania's resources; and (6) determining what steps are necessary to implement the program for the entire school in a way that will not jeopardize the education of current students.

To many members of the university and dental school communities, the major question was the fiscal one: Could the School of Dental Medicine educate its students within a small, personal, private practice environment and still maintain fiscal viability? Could the Model B faculty-based practice be financially viable and if so, what personnel and budgetary requirements would make it so?

In November 1978, the Pew Memorial Trust of the Glenmede Trust Company awarded a grant of $1 million to the University of Pennsylvania School of Dental Medicine to examine these questions by implementing a pilot study based on its Long Range Plan.

The Pennsylvania Experiment would be implemented in the following academic year, 1979–80. The final stages of planning and preparation had to be completed during the less than ten months that remained before the experiment would be fully under way.

Notes

1. Long Range Planning Committee, "Report of the Long Range Planning Committee," January 12, 1977.
2. Ibid. February 1972.
3. Stephen Wotman, "Long Range Planning at the University of Pennsylvania School of Dental Medicine," unpublished paper, 1979.
4. J. T. Dewing and F. K. Foulkes, "University of California at Santa Cruz, Institute for Educational Management, Harvard University," Case 1–372–689 (Boston: Intercollegiate Case Clearing House, 1979).
5. Stephen Wotman, "University of Pennsylvania School of Dental Medicine, Long Range Planning Feasibility Study," November 22, 1977.
6. Martin Meyerson, letter to Dean D. Walter Cohen, January 18, 1978.
7. American Health and Management Corporation, "Assessment of the Market for Dental Services in West Philadelphia and Initial Implications for the School of Dental Medicine's Long Range Plan," May 1978.

4

Design of the Experiment

In November 1978, the School of Dental Medicine faced the task of implementing the Long Range Plan that had resulted from many years of discussion. The Long Range Plan was soon to be known as the Pennsylvania Experiment, a pilot study designed to test the educational and financial concepts and assumptions of the Long Range Planning Committee. To understand the experiment, it is helpful to examine recent models of social science experimentation.

The Pennsylvania Experiment as Reflection-in-Action

Historically, many social scientists have attempted to make social science research conform as closely as possible to the scientific model of experimentation, in which variables are rigorously controlled in the laboratory setting and a great deal of effort goes into obtaining statistically valid and reliable results. In recent years, however, most social scientists have recognized that this model (the "true" experiment) is almost impossible to conform to in the social sciences; the large numbers of confounding variables that occur in human social situations make the true experiment applicable only to the natural sciences. Attempts have therefore been made to adhere to the "quasi experiment," which is essentially a looser, less-controlled form of the true experiment.

Recently social scientists have proposed an altogether different model of experimentation, arguing that even the quasi experiment is unsuitable for social research and furthermore that the true and quasi-experimental models may not be appropriate for the social science experiment. In fact, another model may be better suited to the goals and purposes of social science research. Social intervention experiments, in which planning groups or agencies intervene in the community to effect social change, present an entirely different set of var-

35

iables than other types of research. The social intervention experiment is utilitarian and pragmatic in its purpose; the primary goal of such experiments is usually to improve existing social, educational, and other conditions. They are experimental in that they provide an opportunity to learn by gathering information about what works and what doesn't. Making the experiment work is as important as testing hypotheses, however, because the experiment involves the implementation of a social or educational program.

A newer model of research, reflection-in-action, incorporates many of the concepts embodied in the social intervention experiment. In reflection-in-action,

> the inquirers begin with an initial description of the community situation and an initial framing of the problem they are trying to solve. . . . They predesign only the first round of experimentation. They do not try to hold the conditions of experiment constant, but vary them iteratively throughout the inquiry. They pay attention equally to quantitative data on outcomes and qualitative data on processes of change. They work closely with local practitioners and participants and try to involve them in the tasks of interpretation, analysis and design. They do not try to produce general intervention hypotheses and policy advice; they regard each intervention as a unique case which may become, at best, an exemplar for the design of approaches to other, family-resembling cases. They do not regard the order they observe as an objective pattern of laws inherent in the situation; they recognize that they can test hypotheses only within the bounds of their own ways of describing, framing and transforming the situation. . . . If we view reflection-in-action narrowly, in contrast with the explicit methods of "true" or "quasi" experiment, what stands out is that it brings rapid information feedback, analysis, and redesign of experiment into the intervention itself. In the former models of inquiry, the design of experiment is static and analysis of data is separate from experimental practice; the learning derived from an experiment can only be incorporated in the design of future experiments. In the latter, analysis of data is undertaken in the intervention situation itself and learning from experiment is applied iteratively in the situation to the redesign of the data-gathering system, the experiment, and the strategy of intervention.[1]

The Pennsylvania Experiment can be viewed best within the context of this model. The experiment was not merely an attempt to test educational and financial hypotheses within an isolated, controlled environment; its purpose was to test an innovative approach to dental education in a complex, real-life environment to determine whether this approach could be implemented on a large scale. The social environment of the experiment presented a unique set of variables, which often demanded adjustment and modification of the experimental design. Project administrators worked closely with faculty and students, monitoring the project and redesigning it when necessary. Thus the variables of the experiment were by no means kept constant for three years; if an aspect of the program was not working, it was altered so that the overall curriculum could be tested. The basic principles and the underlying design and structure of the experiment (preceptorship, integrated preclinical and clinical courses, improved student-faculty ratios, fifth-year residency) remained constant throughout the three years of the experiment. Nevertheless, the day-to-day operation of the new program was constantly monitored and modified. In a sense, the evaluation process and the lessons learned started the moment the experiment began. Therefore, it is difficult to divide the experiment into the distinct stages of planning, implementation, and evaluation; the boundaries are much less clear than such a division implies.

At the same time, although this is not a model of the "true" or "quasi" experiment, great effort was given to collecting statistically valid and reliable data. These data were based on objective quantitative measures. The evaluation of the Pennsylvania Experiment had direct consequences for the future of the school; therefore, the evaluation was designed according to the highest standards of systematic evaluation in social science research.

Project Design

The major areas involved in designing the experiment included: faculty and administration recruitment, student recruitment, facilities construction, and curriculum development. In short, a "school within a school" had to be created within ten months, one with little precedent in dental education.

FACULTY AND ADMINISTRATION RECRUITMENT

During the fall of 1978, Dr. Patricia Cormier was selected as educational coordinator to be responsible for developing and overseeing the new curriculum, recruiting students and handling student affairs, and supervising the evaluation of the new program. Dr. Cormier, then assistant professor of Dental Care Systems, had conducted several large-scale community intervention experiments in dental health and brought a strong background in educational psychology and research to the project.

The project administrator was appointed in January 1979. Dr. Alvin Morris, then executive director for the Association of Academic Health Centers in Washington, D.C., had a distinguished background in dental education at the administrative level. He had previously served as dean of the University of Kentucky Dental School and vice-president of the University of Kentucky. With a strong background in innovative approaches to dental education, Dr. Morris was currently involved in the development of fifth-year residency programs. In January 1979, Dr. Morris accepted the School of Dental Medicine's offer to direct the experiment. Unfortunately, he was unable to assume the position until July 1979, so Dr. Cormier served as both educational coordinator and acting director until Dr. Morris's arrival.

The selection of a director for the Model B facility proved to be a difficult task, and a director was not found until March 1979—less than a month before the Model B practice was scheduled to open its doors to patients and well after the construction of its facility was under way. This new position in dental education demanded a rare blend of qualifications. The new director would have to be a master clinician with a strong background in general dentistry and expertise in at least one of the specialties, a proven educator and clinical teacher, a provider with experience and success in private practice management who agreed with the basic concepts of the experiment, and a hard-working, energetic teacher/practitioner/administrator able to weather the challenges of starting a totally new dental practice and educational program at the same time. Providing incentives to attract such a person was difficult. Dentists are essentially entrepreneurial and independent and often do not prefer to work under the aegis of an institution or within a bureaucracy. Indeed, many people are attracted to dentistry precisely because it offers independence and the freedom to be one's own supervisor. This project would demand working closely with administrators. The director of the Model B practice would be taking a risk by leaving a private practice and starting a new one in a different location. Also, Model B had built-in financial limitations; providers would be salaried, whereas in private practice incomes are open-ended and depend on the success of the practice. Above all, this new position promised to be stressful and highly demanding.

In March 1979, after an intensive search, Dr. Robert Tisot was recruited as director of Model B. His qualifications fulfilled all of these requirements. Dr. Tisot had been at the school for fifteen years in a variety of capacities. Starting in the Department of Fixed Prosthetics (now integrated into the Department of Restorative Dentistry), he had moved on to the graduate Department of Periodontics. In 1969, Tisot was selected to direct the clinical phase of an innovative program known as the Committee on Advanced Placement and Accelerated Programs (CAPAP). This program trained students as dentists in three years and then led to either a clinical specialty degree, a Ph.D. in a related field of science, an M.D., an M.B.A., or combinations thereof. As director of this program, Tisot had been given approval by the faculty to certify a student as qualified for graduation in all of the clinical disciplines; he was the only faculty member so qualified. He also had experience in teaching as a preceptor because the program used this model of education. After successfully directing the CAPAP program, Tisot also directed the federally funded Ph.D./D.M.D. training program, which retrained Ph.D.'s in the biological sciences as D.M.D.'s in twenty-four months, giving him additional experience in implementing innovative new programs in dental education. Most recently, Tisot had been clinical director of the program that became the forerunner of the group practices in the main clinic and was director of the general practice residency program, a natural forerunner of the Pennsylvania Experiment with its fifth-year curriculum. In addition, Dr. Tisot had a successful private practice and extensive experience in practice management. In summary, he was a highly respected teacher and master clinician with private practice experience and a strong foundation in some of the key areas of the experiment. In March 1979 he accepted the new position as a master clinician-educator, the first of its kind in dental education.

In March a second clinician-educator was appointed for Model B. Dr. Norman Lurie was an excellent teacher in the main clinic with a strong background in endodontics (complementing Dr. Tisot's expertise in periodontics) and experience as a successful private practitioner.

The director for Model A was also chosen at this time. Dr. Daniel Casullo, a graduate of the Periodontal Prosthesis Program at Penn, brought an excellent background in total dentistry and a commitment to the preceptor model of education to this role. Dr. Casullo had successfully implemented the group practice model in the main clinic and was highly respected for his teaching as well as clinical abilities. He was also a successful private practitioner with a strong commitment to comprehensive dentistry and to an integrated approach to the care of the human dentition.

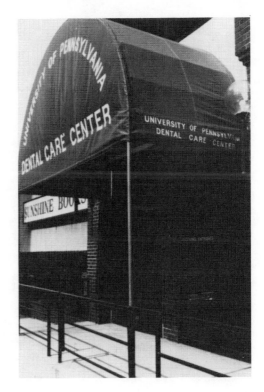

The School built a new health-care facility in 1979, the Dental Care Center, in space rented for this purpose at 4003 Spruce Street.

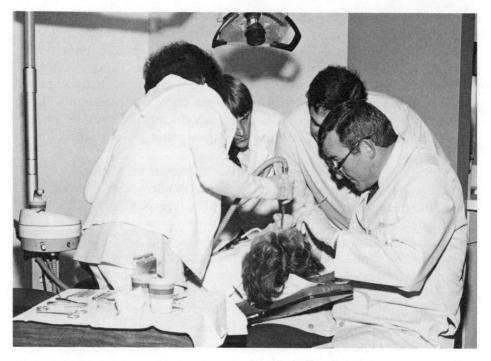

Preceptor demonstrating delivery of oral health care in Model B to preceptees.

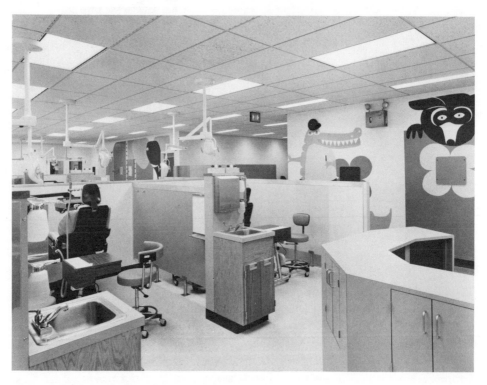

The appointment desk in the Dental Care Center. Model B.

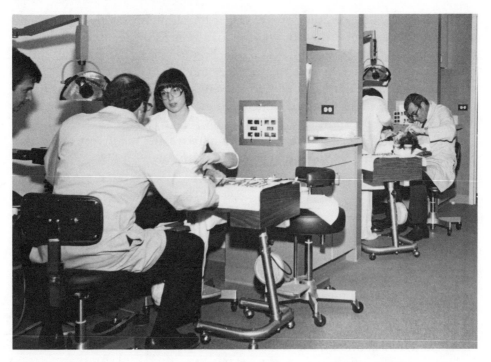

Students learning.

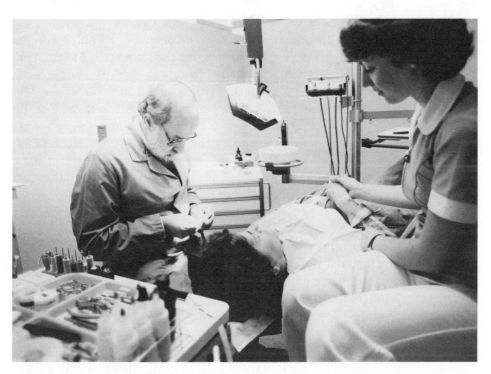

Dr. Robert J. Tisot, Associate Professor of Periodontics and Director of Penn's Dental Care Center.

During April, the selection of a manager for clinic operations was accomplished. Dr. Peter Barnett, a dentist with an advanced degree in business, was hired to oversee the development of clinical protocols, record-keeping, collections, and information systems in Models A and B.

In May five more generalist-educators were selected for Model A, many of whom were preceptees who had worked with Dr. Casullo in the group practice program in the main clinic.

Thus by late spring, the principal administrative and faculty members had been chosen. Additional support staff was hired in August 1979.

FACILITIES

The Kling Partnership architectural firm drew up plans for the Model B facility in the fall of 1978, using the facilities report prepared a year before by Long Range Planning Committee member Dale Wade. What was most essential was that its dual nature as both a private practice facility and an educational facility responsible for the clinical education of students be reflected. Faculty and students would require easy access to one another, and yet patients would expect an environment that was private and professional. The architectural plans were designed to reflect all of these variables.

Construction was begun on the Model B facility in January; it was completed and equipped in the very short time of ninety days, receiving its first patient on April 15, 1979.

The new Model B facility, named the Dental Care Center, is located on the second floor of a shopping center adjacent to the School of Dental Medicine. It is a modern, naturally lit facility. Upon entering the Dental Care Center, one faces a long reception desk, which is staffed by one to three receptionists. In back of the reception area is a large space with several desks, bordered on the rear by filing shelves constructed to hold the patient records. To the rear of this area are several offices, a conference room, and a student lounge. In front of the reception area is a large waiting room, furnished with a low rectangular table bordered on three sides by blue couches and two coffee tables. The furniture is modern, and the waiting area is bright and well-lit. Plants, wall hangings, and paintings decorate the walls and corners of the room. To the left of this reception area, a walkway leads to two double doors, from which the faculty or student provider comes to greet the patient. The patient is led through these doors, to be seated in one of sixteen modern, well-equipped operatories. These operatories are clustered in four groups of four chairs each with an internal corridor running through each group to allow easy access from one operatory to the next. Thus the operatories are private, yet they allow faculty and students to work closely together. Each group of operatories has a large supply area directly adjacent to it, fully stocked and equipped with X-ray machines. In back of these operatories and supply areas is a hallway leading into the student lounge area (located in back of the reception area), equipped with a small kitchen area, tables, and chairs.

On April 15, 1979, the Dental Care Center opened its doors as a faculty private practice, staffed by Dr. Norman Lurie and Dr. Robert Tisot. Several open houses were held during the first month of the practice to introduce the West Philadelphia and university communities to the Dental Care Center. Marketing efforts also included notices in local papers and a mailing to the West Philadelphia community. The Dental Care Center began building slowly as a private practice, with Dr. Tisot's and Dr. Lurie's patients providing a foundation. By September 1979, approximately five to six hundred patients were being seen in the practice.

Construction of Model A, the Paletz Clinic, a fifteen-chair clinic located in the northeast corner of the basement of the Evans Building, was completed during the summer. Like Model B, the operatories in the clinic are arranged to allow easy access among faculty members and students and to facilitate four-handed sit-down dentistry. The preclinical laboratory is directly adjacent to the clinical area, encouraging the integration of clinical and preclinical learning. A waiting area directly outside the clinic provides comfortable seating for patients, as in a private practice, as well as space for several receptionists and an office coordinator.

STUDENT SELECTION

For the first year of the experiment, student selection for all but the incoming first-year class was done by application. Applicants were randomly selected from each quintile of their respective classes (based on grade point average in dental school), to assure that the experiment contained a cross-section of the student body. Seven students from the Classes of 1979, 1980, and 1981 each were selected in this way to participate in the experiment in 1979–80 as residents, seniors, and juniors, respectively. Four students would be in Model A, and three would be in Model B. Ten students were chosen from the Class of 1982 (to be sophomores), six for Model A, and four for Model B.

Incoming first-year students (the Class of 1983) were informed about the experiment when they were sent their acceptance letters to dental school and were asked to check a box if they were interested in the new program. Random selection was then made from each quintile of the group expressing interest (based on undergraduate grade point average) of fourteen students (eight for Model A, six for Model B). (See Appendix VII for a list of all students participating in the Pennsylvania Experiment.)

CURRICULUM

During the spring and summer, Dr. Cormier worked on the design and development of a new curriculum to be implemented in the fall of 1979 for thirty-two students in the Pennsylvania Experiment in all four years of dental school

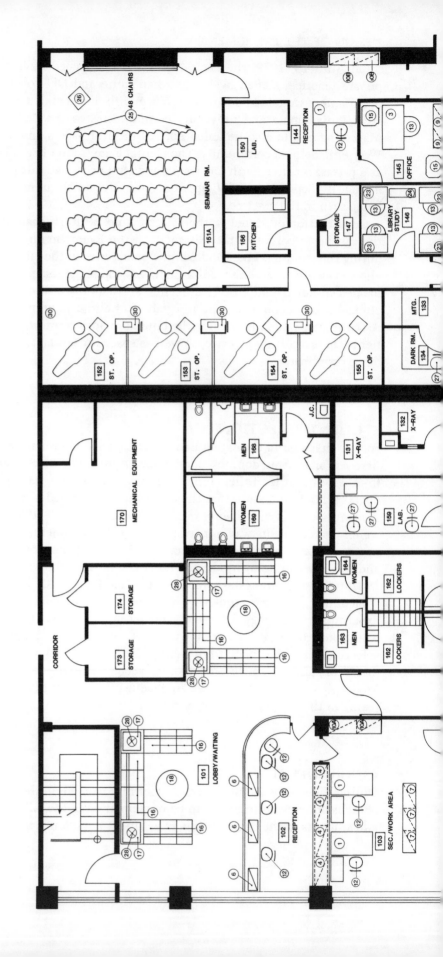

U OF P DENTAL FACILITY-PLAN

OP. 122

OP. 123

OP. 124

OP. 125

137

136 STERILIZATION

135 WORK RM.

160 STORAGE

TYPICAL CORE. & EQUIPMENT

121

OP. 120

OP. 119

OP. 118

OPERATORY

OP. 114

OP. 115

OP. 116

OP. 117

STAFF CORRIDOR

126 DENTISTRY

127 STERILIZATION

128 WORK RM.

160 STORAGE

113

OPERATORY

OP. 112

OP. 111

OP. 110

TYPICAL OPERATORY & EQUIPMENT

104 BUS. MGR.

105 CONF. RM.

106 DENTIST OFF.

108 STAFF LOUNGE

as well as a residency year. Deborah Diserens, an educational consultant, assisted Dr. Cormier in this task.

Some basic framework for the new curriculum had been provided by the eleven recommendations of the Long Range Planning Committee, which had suggested inclusion of the following components: (1) a fifth-year general family practice residency program; (2) the preceptor model of clinical instruction, using preceptor teams; (3) a faculty-based group practice; (4) improved student-faculty ratios; (5) an integrated preclinical technique course; (6) earlier entry into clinical education; (7) an oral biology core sequence; (8) courses in behavioral and social sciences; (9) practice organization and management courses; and (10) the integration of dental auxiliary education with the clinical education of dental students.

Many of these ideas had been discussed and developed further into more concrete plans. The concept of the Model A and Model B clinical sites had been developed during 1976 to 1978 (Model A as a transitional group practice clinic stressing comprehensive care and increased faculty participation in care with improved student-faculty ratios, and Model B as a faculty-based group practice in which faculty both treated patients and educated students).

The curricular outlines were formulated by June 1979 based on this groundwork. The new curriculum was based on a twofold summary of the Long Range Plan:

> It is the fundamental assumption of the Long Range Plan that the dental professional who will be best prepared for the future and who will best serve the population will be that person who:
> (1) has been trained as a general practitioner of dentistry, possessing extended clinical competence and skills so that he or she will be able to perform all but the most complex procedures currently referred to specialists;
> (2) has received a broad-based professional education in fields beyond those currently contained in the dental curriculum, resulting in the graduation of a dentist who possesses a broad understanding of his or her role in society, a belief in the merits of a collaborative approach to health care delivery, a commitment to the humane treatment of patients, and experience and skills in performing clinical teaching.[2]

Figure 4-1 outlines the experimental curriculum, comparing it to the traditional curriculum of the school. The technical skills and knowledge required of the student in the experiment remain identical to those required of the traditional student. Education in the basic sciences, in particular, is identical for both experimental and traditional students. Although some additional material on behavioral sciences and practice management, as well as a fifth-year residency program, have been added to the new curriculum, the content of the undergraduate curriculum remains essentially unaltered. (The addition of a fifth year obviously provides additional educational experiences, and earlier entry into clinical settings allows for accelerated clinical learning.) The Pennsylvania Experiment does change significantly the manner in which the curriculum is organized and presented to students and the environment in which learning takes place.

The major curricular changes included in the experiment are as follows: (1) a new separate course of preclinical education which integrates previously distinct laboratory courses into one unified course taught in a laboratory directly adjacent to the Model A clinical setting (facilitating the understanding of practical applications of techniques). The course is taught by the same faculty who teach the students clinically in Model A and by residents from Models A and B, thereby facilitating continuity and reducing the amount of repetition for students during their clinical years; (2) proximity between the preclinical laboratory and the clinical environment; (3) the inclusion of several new courses in human behavior, interdisciplinary health care, and practice management; (4) earlier student entry into clinical education (beginning in the first year rather than in the third year of dental school); (5) an entirely new environment for clinical education, featuring increased faculty participation in care, improved student-faculty ratios, and a more real-life setting; (6) integration of the specialties in clinical education and more comprehensive care for patients; (7) inclusion of a fifth-year residency program; (8) integration of dental hygiene students (in Model A only) and of dental hygiene providers (in both Models A and B) into the clinical environment in which experimental students are educated, facilitating the use of team dentistry.

Attempts to implement an oral biology course were unsuccessful because of strong objections by certain basic science faculty members to this innovation.

A summary of the curriculum in each year of dental school follows.

First-Year Curriculum

The major change during the freshman year for students in the experiment and the essence of the first-year curriculum is an entirely revised preclinical laboratory course of education. All fourteen first-year students in the experiment participate in this course, which is held in a laboratory located directly adjacent to Model A. The course, designed by Dr. Daniel Casullo and Dr. Daniel Boston with the assistance of Ms. Diserens, integrates the previously separate laboratory courses of operative, orthodontics/pedodontics, and form and function of the masticatory system (FFMS) into one general dentistry laboratory course. The course introduces peer review into the first-year student's experience; each student receives a faculty, self-, and peer evaluation of his/her work in the laboratory. This preclinical curricula is illustrated in Figure 4-2.

Students also participate in a course training them as chairside assistants during the first semester, developed and taught by Dr. Norma Kaplis. Dr. Kaplis, an assistant professor of dental care systems, was formerly the clinical director of a program educating students in team delivery. Students function as chairside dental assistants to a faculty or resident provider in their second se-

Figure 4-1. Pennsylvania Experiment and Traditional Curricula

	First Year	Second Year	Third Year	Fourth Year	Fifth Year
Pennsylvania Experiment	Preclinical general dentistry (lab) Human behavior Chairside dental assisting Preventive dentistry	Anesthesia and pain control (lab) Preclinical general dentistry (lect and lab) Expanded functions dental assisting General dentistry clinical seminar Interdisciplinary health care General dentistry clinic	General dentistry clinic (model A or B)	General dentistry clinic (model A or B) Teaching skills practicum Practice management seminar	General practice residency
Both Groups (Traditional and Experimental)	All basic sciences Dental materials Form and function (lect) Operative (lect) Orthodontics/pedodontics (lect) Dental care systems Radiology (lect)	All basic sciences Orthodontics/pedodontics (lect) Oral medicine (lect) Anesthesia and pain control (lect) Diagnostic radiology (lect)	Form and function (lect) Restorative (lect) Orthodontics/pedodontics Pedodontics (clinic) Adjunctive orthodontics (clinic and lab) Endodontics (lect) Oral medicine (lect) Oral surgery (lect) Periodontics (lect) Training in expanded auxiliary management (lect)	Pedodontic clinic Extramural hospital rotation Selectives	

Figure 4-1. Pennsylvania Experiment and Traditional Curricula (continued)

	First Year	Second Year	Third Year	Fourth Year	Fifth Year
Traditional	Form and function (lab) Operative (lab) Orthodontics/periodontics Dental health education	Form and function (lect and lab) Operative (lect and lab) Fixed prosthetics (lect and lab) Removable prosthetics (lect) Orthodontics/periodontics (lab) Endodontics (lect and lab) Periodontics (lect and lab) Dental auxiliary utilization (lect)	Main clinic (restorative) Removable prosthetics Endodontics clinic Oral medicine clinic Oral surgery clinic Dental auxiliary utilization (lect)	Main clinic (restorative and perio) Removable prosthesis Endodontics clinic Oral medicine clinic Oral surgery clinic	

Figure 4-2. Traditional and Pennsylvania Experiment Preclinical Curricula

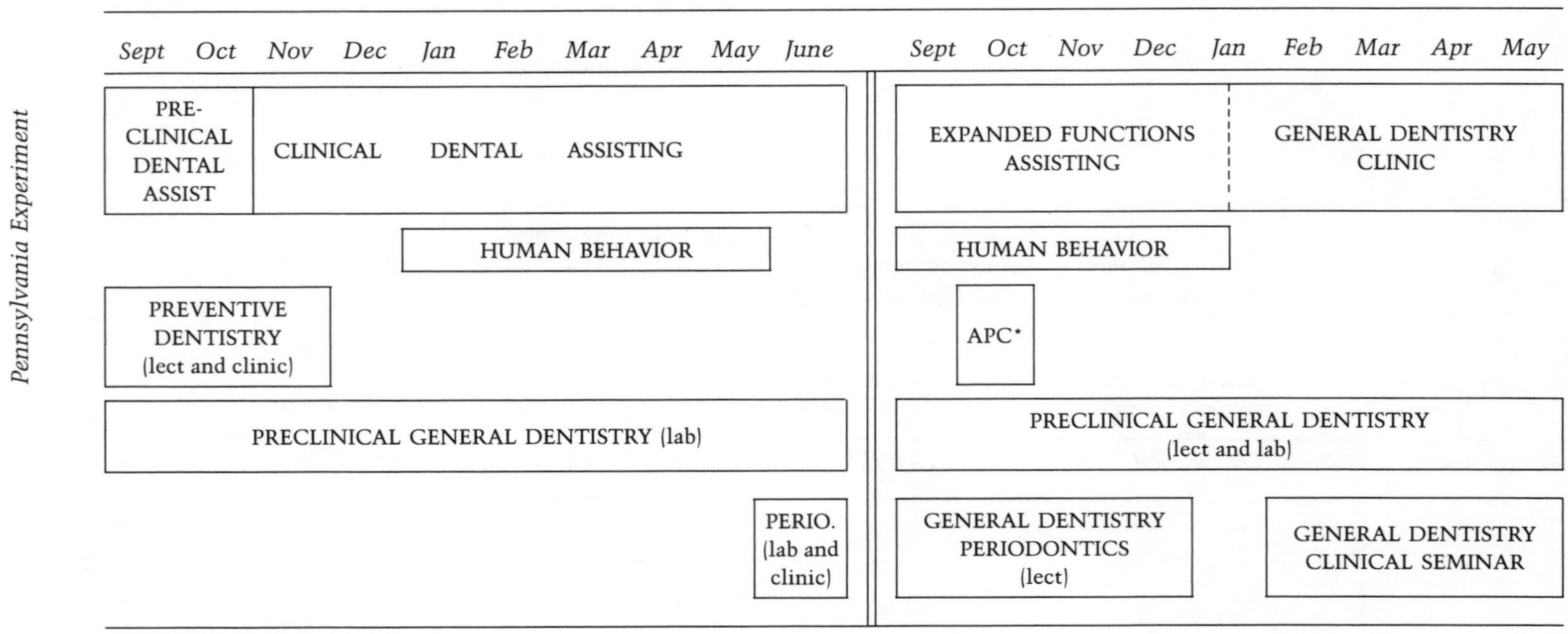

Freshman Year

Sophomore Year

Sept Oct Nov Dec Jan Feb Mar Apr May June | Sept Oct Nov Dec Jan Feb Mar Apr May

PRE-CLINICAL DENTAL ASSIST

CLINICAL DENTAL ASSISTING

EXPANDED FUNCTIONS ASSISTING

GENERAL DENTISTRY CLINIC

HUMAN BEHAVIOR

HUMAN BEHAVIOR

PREVENTIVE DENTISTRY (lect and clinic)

APC*

PRECLINICAL GENERAL DENTISTRY (lab)

PRECLINICAL GENERAL DENTISTRY (lect and lab)

PERIO. (lab and clinic)

GENERAL DENTISTRY PERIODONTICS (lect)

GENERAL DENTISTRY CLINICAL SEMINAR

Pennsylvania Experiment

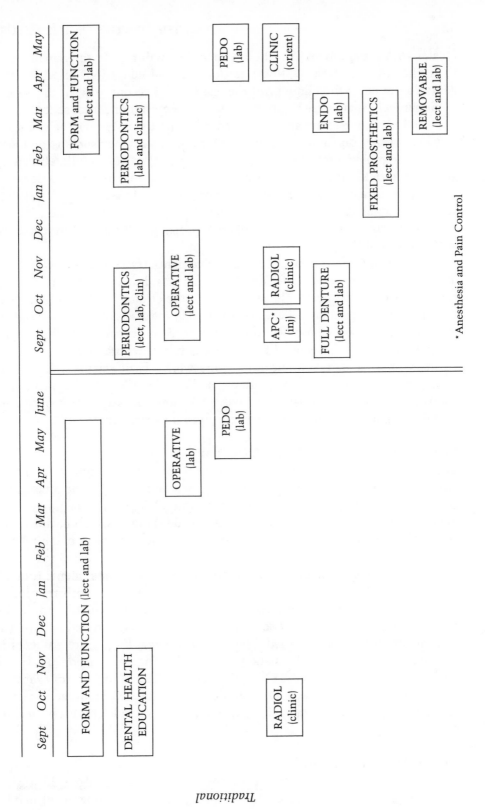

Sophomore Year

Freshman Year

Traditional

FORM and FUNCTION (lect and lab)

PEDO (lab)

CLINIC (orient)

PERIODONTICS (lab and clinic)

ENDO (lab)

REMOVABLE (lect and lab)

FIXED PROSTHETICS (lect and lab)

PERIODONTICS (lect, lab, clin)

OPERATIVE (lect and lab)

RADIOL (clinic)

APC* (inj)

FULL DENTURE (lect and lab)

Sept Oct Nov Dec Jan Feb Mar Apr May

*Anesthesia and Pain Control

Sept Oct Nov Dec Jan Feb Mar Apr May June

FORM AND FUNCTION (lect and lab)

DENTAL HEALTH EDUCATION

OPERATIVE (lab)

PEDO (lab)

RADIOL (clinic)

mester within the model (A or B) in which they will receive the remainder of their clinical education. Unlike traditional dental education, in which students do not enter the clinic until the end of their second year, in the experiment clinical experiences begin with the first semester of dental school.

Several new courses are also presented in the first year. Human behavior is a series of twenty one-and-one-half-hour seminars on topics such as problem-solving and problem ownership, listening skills, anger, how to talk effectively, giving feedback, intervention strategies, building relationships, leadership styles, participative management and motivation, role analysis, professional values, personal values, and interviewing. Experiential exercises are included in these seminars, taught by Dr. Robert Emling, an educational psychologist at the School of Dental Medicine.

A twenty-eight-hour course in preventive dentistry consisting of thirteen lectures and seven two-hour clinical sessions was developed. The purpose of this course is to familiarize the student with the etiology and pathogenesis of dental caries and periodontal disease, to develop the skills of daily oral hygiene implementation, and above all, to help the student develop a preventive philosophy as the daily basis of a lifelong successful dental practice.

First-year students take their other coursework—basic sciences, dental materials, radiology, dental care systems, and the lectures for the preclinical course—with traditional students. Figure 4-3 shows the sequencing of courses in the freshman curriculum of the Pennsylvania Experiment.

GOALS OF THE FIRST-YEAR CURRICULUM
The goals of the first-year curriculum are to (1) present students with an integrated course in the preclinical sciences to include training in the preparation and restoration of the form and function of normal dentition, diagnosis, treatment planning, and therapy of caries; (2) provide training which begins to develop in students an understanding of the collaborative delivery of dental care in a group practice setting and to provide opportunities for students to interact with all members of the dental care delivery team and with students from all four classes within the clinical setting; (3) provide students with training in communications and human interaction skills and an introduction to the application of the behavioral sciences in dental care; (4) train students to use the mechanism of peer review in the preclinical setting; (5) prepare students to function as chairside dental assistants; (6) prepare students to record a patient's medical history and take vital signs; (7) prepare students to perform examinations of the oral soft tissues and the head and neck; (8) reinforce students' radiographic techniques; and (9) prepare students to provide clinical preventive dentistry.

Second-Year Curriculum
The sophomore year curriculum continues along the lines begun during the first year, presenting an integrated preclinical program including the principles

Figure 4-3. Sequencing of Courses in the Freshman Curriculum of the Pennsylvania Experiment

Content Areas

Weeks			
1	General Dentistry Lab: (Anatomy and Restorative)	Preclinical Dental Assisting	General Dentistry Preventive Dentistry (Lecture)
2			
3	Add-on waxing		
4	Dental anatomy projects		
5	Occlusion landmark relationships		
6			
7			
8	Restoration of toothform		Clinical Preventive Dentistry
9			
10		Clinical Dental Assisting	
11			
12			
13	Class I amalgam preparations		
14			
15	Class II amalgam preparations		
16	EXAMS		
17–18	Christmas Break		

Figure 4-3. Sequencing of Courses in the Freshman Curriculum of the Pennsylvania Experiment (continued)

Content Areas

Weeks

Week	
19	Class V amalgam preparations
20	
21	Extensive amalgam preparations
22	
23	Class III amalgam preparations
24	
25	Pedodontic preparations
26	
27	DFG preparations and restorations
28	
29	Spring Break
30	Composite restorations
31	Inlay preparations
32	
33	
34	Functional occlusion
35	
36	Single tooth cast restorations
37	
38	EXAMS
39	Summer Break
40	
41	
44	

Human Behavior

General Dentistry
Periodontics
Preclinical Lab

and techniques of basic periodontics, operative dentistry, endodontics, pediatric dentistry, full and partial dentures, and fixed prosthetics, all taught in one course offered in the preclinical laboratory of Model A. In the second year, both laboratory work and lectures are offered in the experimental setting (in contrast to the first-year course, which offers preclinical labs only in a separate environment). The course is guided by generalist-educators, residents from Models A and B, and consulting specialists.

Students' early exposure to clinical training continues, with a didactic course in expanded functions dental assisting given by Dr. Kaplis in the first semester, followed by clinical exposure to patient care in the second semester (diagnosis and treatment planning, radiographs, periodontal procedures, and some operative procedures).

Separate courses are given in anesthesia and pain control, interdisciplinary health care, and, during the first year of the experiment, human behavior (because sophomore students did not receive the course as freshmen). As in the first-year curriculum, all basic science lectures are taken with the rest of the student body. See Figure 4-4 for the sequencing of courses in the sophomore curriculum.

GOALS OF THE SECOND-YEAR CURRICULUM

The goals of the second-year curriculum are to (1) provide opportunities for students to interact with all members of the dental care delivery team and with students of all levels within the clinical setting; (2) present students with an integrated course in the preclinical sciences to include occlusion, endodontics, fixed and removable prosthesis, and periodontics; (3) provide students with the opportunity to participate in the clinical setting as expanded function dental assistants; (4) provide beginning clinical experience for students in restorative dentistry; (5) provide additional opportunities for students to record a patient's medical history and take vital signs; (6) provide additional opportunities for students to perform examinations of the oral soft tissues and the head and neck; (7) provide additional preclinical experiences for students in anesthesia and pain control; (8) provide opportunities for students to perform periodontal therapy, to include scaling and root planing.

Third- and Fourth-Year Curriculum

During the third and fourth years, the clinical training of students intensifies. It is during these years that students experience what is perhaps the single most important aspect of the experiment: a totally new environment and approach to clinical education. Students spend all of their clinical time, with the exception of two rotations into pedodontics and oral surgery (and hospital rotations for residents), in either Model A or Model B. To understand this key aspect of the experiment, it is helpful to examine the traditional clinical setting at the school.

The main clinic at the school is the site where all third- and fourth-year

Figure 4-4. Sequencing of Courses in the Sophomore Curriculum of the Pennsylvania Experiment

Content Areas

Weeks			
1	General Dentistry (Restorative Endodontics and Occlusion)	Expanded Functions Dental Assisting	General Dentistry Periodontics Lecture
2			
3	Amalgam preparation and restoration review		
4	Porcelain jacket crowns		Preclinical Local Anesthesia
5			
6	Pedodontics		
7			
8	Fixed partial dentures		
9			
10			
11			
12			
13			
14	Endodontics		
15			
16	EXAMS		
17	Christmas Break		

Content Areas

Weeks

Weeks	Content Areas
18	Post/core
19	Parapost
20	Removable partial dentures
21	
22	
23	
24	
25	Full dentures
26	
27	
28	
29	Spring Break
30	Occlusion and occlusal appliances
31	
32	
33	
34	
35	
36	
37	
38	EXAMS
39	Summer Break
40	
41	
42	

General Dentistry Clinical Seminar

General Dentistry Clinical Practice

Human Behavior

clinical students receive their clinical education. It is a vast room, containing 136 chairs grouped in bays of 12 chairs each. The chairs are lined up near one another, without any separating devices. Clinical protocols demand that students wait in line for supplies (which they can obtain only after receiving a cashier's receipt for their patient's payments). These procedures are designed to control the flow of supplies. The student-faculty ratio is approximately 12:1. Students treat their patients according to a predetermined sequence, which constitutes their clinical curriculum. Contrary to dental practice, students take their patients into five separate clinics for their various dental needs. Because no faculty or resident providers practice in the clinic, cases are restricted to those that can be completed successfully by predoctoral dental students. The clinic gives students no exposure to the realities of dental practice or practice management.

By contrast, students in the Pennsylvania Experiment receive their clinical education in an entirely different environment—one that is more closely aligned to the dental environment they will face after graduation. Furthermore, the setting is one which they have been exposed to from their first year of dental school; therefore, transition into the clinic in the third year is much smoother and more efficient than is often the case in traditional dental education. The large clinical setting is replaced by Model A or Model B, in which students provide comprehensive care in restorative dentistry (operative, crown and bridge, full and partial dentures, periodontics, endodontics, preventive dentistry, and oral diagnosis and treatment planning).

Model A is a small fifteen-chair clinic, which, unlike the main clinic, has residents, dental hygiene students, and dental hygiene providers in addition to third-, fourth-, and some second- and first-year students. The student-faculty ratio is 5:1, and faculty have increased participation in patient care and more responsibility and accountability for patient care than in the traditional setting. Students have the advantage of studying clinically under the same faculty members who taught them preclinically. Model A functions far more like an actual practice (they do not have to stand in line for supplies, and a receptionist schedules appointments and collects patient fees). Because of the presence of residents, it receives more advanced cases for treatment and has a wider population base than that seen in the main clinic (particularly a larger proportion of older patients). The Model A clinic emphasizes comprehensive dental care using both generalist and specialist faculty members in an integrated setting. Integration of auxiliaries in the team approach (multihanded, sit-down dentistry) is also used. Rotations are made only to oral surgery and pedodontics with all other care taking place in one setting.

Model A also uses vertical groups to facilitate the preceptor model of education. Students are assigned to groups containing first-, second-, third-, and fourth-year students, residents, and faculty members. This system facilitates the development of teaching skills in residents and upper-class students and helps to assure that students receive adequate attention.

Model B functions as a private group practice in a modern, well-furnished and equipped private practice facility. Eventually, three receptionists, one insurance clerk, a data input clerk, and an office manager staffed the practice. Because it is a private practice run by master clinicians, students are exposed to a large, complex range of cases, as well as a large patient base that more closely matches that seen in the environment outside of dental school. In addition, students treat patients on third-party payment programs. Students work closely with faculty as coproviders and coprofessionals and use the team approach with the trained dental assistants and auxiliaries on staff. As in Model A, they are placed in vertical groups, which include faculty providers, residents, and fourth- and third-year students in each group, with each student assigned to specific residents and faculty members.

Students from Model B rotate to Model A for their pedodontic training and, as do Model A students, they rotate to the main dental school for one session of oral surgery. (Oral surgery procedures are done in both models; this rotation is performed primarily to satisfy the graduation requirements of the traditional program.) Comprehensive care is emphasized, and students are the beneficiaries of a greatly improved student-faculty ratio (4:1).

Faculty in Model B have full income responsibility and complete participation in patient care. The Dental Care Center uses a problem-oriented patient record to facilitate peer review in the clinical setting. Both clinical settings have clinical seminars one or two times a week in their respective models, facilitating student presentation of cases and peer review.

Fourth-year students in both models also receive additional classes in practice management and teaching skills.

GOALS OF THIRD- AND FOURTH-YEAR CURRICULUM

The goals of the third and fourth years are to (1) provide the students with training in the delivery of comprehensive, integrated care in an environment that will foster attention to individual students and encourage students to progress clinically as rapidly as their skill warrants, especially in the areas of periodontics, crown and bridge, endodontics, and operative dentistry; (2) provide students with experience in and understanding of the collaborative delivery of dental care through (a) the integration of students and providers, (b) clinical training in a group practice setting, and (c) weekly treatment planning seminars; (3) further students' understanding of the factors influencing the interaction between dentist and patient and among dental colleagues, as well as auxiliaries; and (4) provide fourth-year students with an opportunity to teach preclinical techniques and guide first- and second-year students who serve as chairside assistants in the clinic.

Fifth-Year Curriculum

Students remain in the clinical setting in which they received their previous education (A or B) for their fifth year and also spend one-third of their time in a hospital setting.

The fifth-year program presents extensive academic and clinical coursework in endodontics, operative dentistry, oral surgery, orthodontics, pedodontics, periodontics, prosthodontics, and physical evaluation. The curriculum stresses the development of treatment-planning skills and the integration of the specialties into a system of overall dental care. The academic program is taught by Model A faculty, and the clinical teaching takes place in the models. Students also receive exposure to a wide range of clinical settings, including several major urban hospitals (Veterans Administration Hospital, Medical College of Pennsylvania, Graduate Hospital, and Einstein Medical Center).

The teaching program is a key aspect of the fifth-year curriculum; students are assigned one day of teaching responsibilities per week, both in the preclinical laboratories and within their clinical settings as members of a vertical group. In addition, a seminar series covers topics related to teaching such as problem-solving and teaching, conditions, types, and motivation for learning, and personality and external influences on students.

An extensive peer review program gives students direct experience in the techniques and methods of quality assurance. Students perform peer review evaluations of one another, using a set of criteria agreed upon by all participants. Students' diagnostic, clinical, and interpersonal skills are considered. This program is complemented by a lecture series covering topics such as state of the art in quality assurance and financial viability, assuring quality among employees and giving feedback, and deriving a workable model of peer review. Other features of the curriculum include journal clubs and seminars in literature review, care for the medically compromised patient, communication skills, and practice management.

GOALS OF RESIDENCY PROGRAM
The goals of the residency program are to develop in students (1) understanding of prevention, diagnosis, treatment planning, and total patient care; (2) competence and confidence in the various dental disciplines which are an integral part of general dentistry; (3) understanding of an integrated, multidisciplinary approach to therapy; (4) ability to make judgments (clinical problem-solving, academic problem-solving, and fiscal problem-solving); (5) ability to interact effectively with all health practitioners as well as with patients; (6) understanding of the principles of education and experience in teaching in preclinical programs; (7) understanding of the consideration and skills involved in treating all age groups; (8) academic experience through reviewing scholarly papers, preparing and giving lectures, and studying the current literature; (9) understanding of factors affecting both the financial and personnel management of a dental practice; (10) understanding of quality assurance in dentistry, with particular emphasis on the development and implementation of a system of peer review.

In August 1979, an in-service training was held for faculty in the experiment to orient them to the new curriculum. In September 1979, the Pennsylvania Experiment went into full operation for all five classes of students and residents.

Notes

1. D. A. Schon, W. Drake, and R. Miller, "Social Experimentation as Reflection-in-Action: Community Level Nutrition Intervention Revisited," November 1982, unpublished paper.
2. *The Busch Center Report on the Pennsylvania Experiment, 1980–82*, Vol. I, University of Pennsylvania School of Dental Medicine, unpublished report.

5

Implementation

The Pennsylvania Experiment was implemented during academic year 1979–80 and ran for three consecutive years.

Preclinical Program (Freshman and Sophomore)

As indicated in Chapter 4, the experiment featured a separate integrated preclinical general dentistry laboratory course and a didactic chairside assisting course (followed by weekly experiences in chairside assisting) for the freshman class. In the first year, fourteen first-year students participated in these courses, eight who had been assigned to Model A and six who would receive their clinical education in Model B. The experimental freshman curriculum was accelerated and intensive; freshmen students took a total of 353 more clock hours of coursework during the first year than their traditional counterparts.

The preclinical laboratory course was held directly adjacent to the Model A laboratory. Faculty included Model A generalists and fifth-year students from Models A and B. The course fostered a sense of closeness and camaraderie among students, largely because of the smallness of the group and the excellent student-faculty ratio. (Fourteen students were instructed by one of several generalist-educators from Model A.) Many students later reported in interviews that the group was unusually close-knit and supportive and that honesty and trust of one another rather than competitiveness were valued and rewarded by the group. Faculty-student relations seemed friendlier and less formal than in the traditional program. As part of the laboratory course and while assisting chairside, students often saw cases in the adjacent Model A clinic which illustrated the techniques being taught in the preclinical laboratory, giving them immediate clinical exposure to procedures being learned preclinically. Peer review functioned successfully in the laboratories; students received self-, peer, and instructor evaluations.

During the second semester of the first year, all students took an additional course in human behavior, to which they responded enthusiastically. The evaluation of the experiment later demonstrated that this course had a significant impact on students' interpersonal skills (see Chapter 6). Freshman students took all other courses (basic science lectures) with their classmates in the traditional program.

During the first year of the experiment (1979–80), sophomore students continued their preclinical course in the traditional program which they had begun as freshmen. The only difference in the sophomore curriculum was a didactic course in expanded dental functions, including placement and carving of amalgam restorations, placement and finishing of composites, basic periodontal therapy, and chairside assisting functions. By Year II of the experiment (1980–81), a separate second-year preclinical course had been developed for the sophomore class, including both preclinical laboratories and lectures. Because of the intensive preparation in the first-year preclinical course, sophomore students in Years II and III of the experiment required less preclinical lecture time than did sophomores in the traditional program. These students therefore had more clinical time.

MODEL A

Year I (1979–1980)

Model A was the site of the clinical education of four residents, four fourth-year students, four third-year students, six second-year students, eight first-year students, and ten dental hygiene students during the first year of the experiment. One director and ten part-time faculty members (totaling four full-time equivalent [FTE] educators), one full-time dental hygiene faculty member, and four dental assistants supervised the clinical education of these students and residents.

First- and second-year students participated in chairside dental assisting and expanded functions, respectively, during the second semester, being assigned to a vertical group consisting of a faculty member, resident, fourth-year, and third-year students. Freshman students assisted residents, fourth-, and sometimes third-year students in their vertical group.

Residents, juniors, and seniors assigned to Model A had their entire clinical education in the Paletz Clinic in the first year of the project. The clinic used a two-tiered payment schedule, with higher fees being charged by residents than by students. Fees for Model A students were comparable to those of students in both the traditional and Model B programs. The Paletz Clinic was in some ways similar to the main clinic of the traditional program, but in other ways it was quite different. The Paletz Clinic is located in the basement of the main (Evans) building, near the rest of the dental school. But whereas the main clinic has 136 operatories, there are only 15 chairs in the Paletz Clinic. The equipment is modern and suitable for multihanded sit-down dentistry. Faculty educators assume an extended role in treatment. Although they do not treat their own patients in the clinic (as in Model B), they have extended responsibility and accountability for patient treatment, and they perform hands-on dentistry as preceptor/teachers. The presence of faculty as well as residents, dental hygiene faculty, and dental assistants lends a wider range of skills and experience to the clinic. Shortly after the Paletz Clinic was established, it became a major recipient of patient referrals from the main clinic. Advanced cases of dental disease as well as disabled and elderly patients were frequently referred to Model A. In July 1980, an emergency service was added to the clinic, further establishing it as a place to which main clinic patients were referred.

The Paletz Clinic progressed well in its first year. After one full year of operation (by September 1980), it was ahead of its target for total revenues (achieving 34 percent of its fiscal year 1980 targets at the 25 percent point). Particularly promising after the first year were the data on resident and fourth-year student productivity, which appeared to be significantly higher than national averages.

Several problem areas surfaced during the first year of the clinic's operation. These included controlling supply costs and collecting patient payments. As mentioned previously, collection of payments in the main clinic of the dental school is assured because students are required to present cashier's receipts before receiving supplies for treatment. By contrast, in both Models A and B, collections are handled by a receptionist at the front desk as they are in other private practices or clinics. Even in a private practice, however, the collection process must be facilitated by the provider, who either escorts the patient to the front desk after treatment or mentions the payment procedure during the patients' visits. The students in Model A had little experience in collecting payments and had been given little exposure to this area of practice management; thus they often allowed the patients to leave without mentioning payment. Therefore, collection of fees was a problem during the initial stages of the experiment.

In the main clinic, laboratory charges are controlled by a system which requires receipts for payments and demands. Students receive supplies and equipment by retrieving them from a central supply area. By contrast, in Model A there were limited controls over supplies. Also, students were working with more advanced cases than those seen in the main clinic. These two factors resulted in another problem—excessively high laboratory charges during Year I.

Years II and III (1980–1981 and 1981–1982)
During the second year of the experiment (1980–81), six residents, six fourth-year students, six third-year students, eight second-year students, eight first-year students, and nine dental hygiene students were educated clinically in Model A. In Year III (1981–82) eight residents, eight fourth-year students, eight third-year students, eight second-year students, eight first-year students, and ten dental hygiene students spent their clinical time in the model. During the

third year, a dental hygiene resident was added to the practice as part of the first dental hygiene residency program in the United States. Also at the end of the second year, the model underwent a major administrative change: Dr. Daniel Casullo left his position as director of the clinic to direct the residency program in Model A and was replaced by Dr. Uri Hangorsky, formerly a faculty specialist in periodontics in Model A.

By the second and third years, it became apparent that a "farm system" was beginning to take shape. Two of the six Model A fifth-year students in Year II (1980–81) chose to stay on as faculty members in Model A. Two Model B fifth-year students became Model A faculty in the following year (1981–82). Students reared within the preceptor system felt positive enough about the system that they chose to become a part of it as preceptor/faculty members. (This trend has continued and become even more dramatic: in 1982–83, four out of eight Model A fifth-year students remained in Model A as faculty, and a fifth-year student became a faculty member in the main clinic at the school.) A similar trend had occurred in the Periodontal Prosthesis Program, from which many students assumed faculty positions within the school. Many faculty members and administrators considered this trend to be promising because it offered a solution to the problem of finding qualified, highly competent generalist faculty for the models. It seemed that the future of Model A (and as we will see later, Model B) lay in the rearing of students who would choose to practice in this environment.

The vertical groups also were working successfully. This system facilitated continuity of care; graduating fifth-year students prepared their preceptees (fourth- and third-year students in their vertical groups) to assume responsibility for unfinished cases.

By the end of the experiment, Model A had developed its own distinctive characteristics as a clinic. As mentioned above, it received referrals of advanced cases of dental disease from the traditional main clinic, as well as cases involving geriatric and medically compromised patients. Increased faculty participation and the presence of residents allowed for extensive treatment and more sophisticated treatment planning. The principles of periodontal prosthesis and other advanced specialty techniques, which were rarely used in the traditional main clinic, were often used in Model A, exposing students to a wide range of treatment. The Paletz Clinic had become a sophisticated student clinic featuring excellent facilities and the most advanced treatment. (A detailed description of the service mix and productivity in Model A is provided in Chapter 6).

MODEL B

Year I (1979–1980)

During the first year of the experiment (1979–80), Model B was the site of the clinical education of three residents, three fourth-year students, and three third-year students, as well as four second-year and six first-year students. Model B was staffed by 2.5 FTE master clinicians and three specialists, covering the areas of periodontics, endodontics, and prosthodontics. During the second half of the first year (March 1980), a third master clinician was added—Dr. Arthur Straussberg, who had been a successful practitioner following his graduation from the School of Dental Medicine twenty-five years earlier.

The Model B practice grew steadily in its first year. Beginning with only twenty patients when it opened its doors in April 1979, by November the Dental Care Center was seeing almost a thousand patients, with approximately one hundred new patients being added per month. The practice features a three-tiered payment schedule, with the highest fees being charged by faculty providers, followed by resident fees (equivalent to those of residents in Model A) and student fees (equivalent to student fees in both Model A and the traditional program).

The vertical groupings of students and faculty within Model B were not strictly adhered to after a few months of experimentation; students tended to use faculty members or residents of their choice, based on factors such as accessibility and the needs of patients. Nevertheless, the operatory assignments remained such that each pair of operatory groupings had faculty providers, residents, and third- and fourth-year students functioning with easy access to one another.

The preceptor/preceptee model of education had several features in actual practice. At times, students would sit chairside and formally observe an entire procedure performed by the master clinician, often assisting him or her. Faculty appointment books were available for this purpose so that students could sign up to observe specific procedures. Faculty members or preceptors also made suggestions as to which procedures the student should observe. Preceptorship functioned more informally as well. Students or preceptees often were given the opportunity to observe part of a procedure performed by a faculty member/preceptor. The practitioner would then verbally explain what had preceded the procedure. Students also received direct assistance from faculty members when they needed advice or help in treating their own patients. During "down" (nontreatment) time, another aspect of the preceptor model became apparent: students often had the opportunity to hear faculty members discuss particular cases, thereby gaining increased exposure to various aspects of treatment. The preceptor model was enhanced by the presence of several master clinicians, giving students exposure to different styles of treatment and patient care. Model B also featured regular weekly evening meetings, in which students presented cases, giving them experience in case presentation and, again, increasing their exposure to a variety of treatment methods.

Some of the problems encountered in Model B during its first year of operation were similar to those faced in Model A, such as collection of patient fees. Students and residents were not well trained in this area and often neglected to facilitate payment. Even faculty providers, who had experience in private practice, tended to neglect the collection issue, perhaps because they now were functioning as educators as well as practitioners, within a setting that was concerned as much with dental education as with patient treatment. The transfer of certain components of private practice into the new setting was not always automatic. Also, Model B was a large private practice with sixteen and later twenty dental operatories. In a small dental or medical office, payment is often facilitated because the scale of the practice is small so a patient is unlikely to leave without paying. Collections did not proceed as easily in Model B as they might have in a smaller practice.

Another difficulty associated with the development of Model B involved the clear definition of administrative and managerial roles. As a university-based practice functioning under a project grant, Model B was under the close supervision of the project administration. In a dental practice, administration and management of the practice is generally accomplished by the principal practitioner. Thus a natural conflict existed between project administration and Dental Care Center staff. After some deliberation, it was decided that the director of Model B (Dr. Tisot) would assume responsibility for assigning the duties of all personnel consistent with the goals and requirements of the experiment, the evaluation of job performance of all personnel, scheduling all patient care and educational activities, maintenance and appropriate use of all equipment and the physical facilities of the Dental Care Center, and maintaining the inventory of all supplies at the center.

Years II and III (1980–1981 and 1981–1982)

Years II and III of the Pennsylvania Experiment witnessed the maturing of Model B into a highly successful and unique private practice. During Year II, three residents, four fourth-year, four third-year, four second-year, and four first-year students were in Model B. In Year III, four residents, four fourth-year, four third-year, four second-year, and four first-year students constituted the student population in Model B. The number of full-time generalist faculty increased to four in Year II. Drs. Robert Rose and Jeffrey Pearlman Storch, who had been residents in Model B during the first year of the experiment, became faculty providers in the practice. Dr. Straussberg left the practice and was replaced by a succession of practitioners who remained for varying lengths of time. In addition, Model B was staffed by eight trained dental assistants, three dental hygiene providers, one dental hygiene resident, one insurance clerk, one data input clerk, and one office manager.

PENN FACULTY PRACTICE PLAN

In July 1981 an event occurred that was to have major impact on the Model B practice. At this time the practice experienced an influx of patients which continued through the next several years, transforming the Dental Care Center from a slowly growing private practice into one that soon would be forced to expand its facilities. This influx was the result of a major achievement of project staff in 1980–81: the development of the Penn Faculty Practice Plan (FPP), a capitated dental benefit for faculty and staff of the university.

In 1980 the vice-president for budget and finance at the university requested that the School of Dental Medicine develop a dental benefit for its approximately six thousand employees. Subsequently, Drs. Cormier and Barnett developed a dual-option plan, which would give employees the option of receiving care from a provider of their choice to be covered under an indemnity plan underwritten by Prudential Insurance Company or of receiving care under a capitated plan at the Model B Dental Care Center.

The plan was accepted by the university in March 1981. Aggressive marketing efforts were then launched to introduce the plan to the staff of the university. Open enrollments were held for the plan in April, and on July 1, 1981, the Dental Care Center began accepting patients on the plan.

The new dental care program was received enthusiastically by university staff; by the end of the first year of its implementation, 38 percent of the university family was being served at the Dental Care Center, accounting for a substantial portion of its patient population. Forty-seven percent of the Dental Care Center's new patients in fiscal year 1982 were Penn Faculty Practice Plan patients, and 42 percent of its total visits in that year were from plan patients.

All full-time faculty and staff personnel of the university who have completed one continuous year of service are eligible for the Penn Faculty Practice Plan; when they have completed three years of continuous full-time service their family members become eligible. The cost of coverage for the employee is fully furnished by the university; some contribution is necessary to enroll family members. If the staff or faculty member elects to choose the Penn Faculty Practice Plan (rather than being covered by the Prudential Plan) he or she must receive all care at the Dental Care Center. The plan provides first dollar coverage (i.e., no deductible), and a copayment structure is used, whereby the patient pays a certain percentage of care depending on the treatment provided. Table 5-1 delineates the copayment figures by type of service provided.

Primarily because of the success of the Penn Faculty Practice Plan, in the third year of the experiment an additional four-chair clinic, the Crossman Clinic, was added to the existing Model B facility, making it a twenty-chair practice. As of June 30, 1982, there were 6,600 in the active patient pool.

Other Developments

During Year III, several students in Model B expressed interest in remaining in the practice to teach and practice. Thus as in Model A, the beginnings of a "farm system" were occurring. Students educated in Model B were choosing to continue their careers in this educational environment. As in Model A, it seemed that the future of a practice based on the Model B plan lay in the rearing of students who would choose to practice in such an environment.

Students in Model B also displayed an unusually high sense of commitment

Table 5-1. Comparison of Benefits, Pennsylvania Faculty Practice Plan

Services	Indemnity Benefits Plan (Prudential)	Benefits Plan, Model B Dental Care Center
Preventive and diagnostic	100%	100%
Simple restorative (no lab)	90%	100%
Endodontics	80%	90%
Periodontics	80%	90%
Oral surgery	100%	100%
Major restorative (with lab)	50%	60%
Individual calendar year Maximum coverage for nonorthodontic service	$1,000	None
Orthodontics	50%	50%
Individual lifetime maximum coverage	$1,000	None

and dedication. Often, students and residents chose to work well beyond the normal work-day hours as well as on weekends. Many faculty members and students also noted a high level of enthusiasm about dental school among Model B students and residents. (See Chapter 8 for further discussion.)

At the same time, Model B continued to experience some of the problems mentioned above. Furthermore, a new dimension was added to the collection problem with the advent of the Penn Faculty Practice Plan. Much, if not all, of a patient's payments were covered by the plan, thereby ensuring that a certain percentage of payments would be collected automatically. Therefore, providers, residents, and students tended to be less concerned about patient payments because these payments often consisted of small amounts.

Another problem that had become apparent by Year III was related to the issue of university personnel regulations. As a practice functioning under the aegis of the university, the Dental Care Center was required to comply with its regulations. Salaries and benefits had to be consistent with university standards. This became a problem in several respects. The common practice of putting one's best dental assistant on the front desk was unworkable in Model B, since under personnel regulations the salary of a dental assistant is higher than that of a front desk person (and "promotion" to the front desk would have resulted in a lower salary). Also, the liberal benefits provided by the university, including extensive vacation time, are not suitable for a dental practice. Although the university for the most part can afford to be understaffed during slower periods such as the summer months, a dental practice requires full staffing almost all of the year. Therefore, one of the problems experienced at the Dental Care Center was the high vacation allowance allotted to staff, resulting in understaffing during some periods. These problems are a natural result of having a practice within a larger institutional setting and remain as challenges to be solved in future practice/educational units.

OVERALL PROJECT DEVELOPMENTS, YEAR I

The National Advisory Board (see Appendix IV), composed of major figures in the areas of dental practice, research, and education, met three times during the first two years of the experiment: in June 1980, November 1980, and September 1981. During these meetings the board reviewed the progress of the experiment from its inception through its development. In March 1980 an application was submitted and accepted to extend the project grant for an additional two years, through a grant of $1,932,940, so that the experiment could be evaluated after it had been in full operation for two years following the first (developmental) year.

Clinical-Educator Track

In March 1980 a revised proposal for the clinical-educator track was submitted to the Faculty Senate of the School of Dental Medicine for its approval. This track would allow the clinician-educator to have a secure career path. The clinical-educator track requires that faculty members reach associate professorship in ten years; if they achieve this level, they may then stay on the faculty as long as they continue to generate their salary by means of patient care income. Excerpts from this proposal follow.

According to the proposal,

> There shall be established a category of full-time clinician-educators, who are members of the standing faculty of the University on a non-tenured clinical-educator track, to take effect on July 1, 1980, or as soon thereafter as is administratively practical. These persons are members of the standing faculty of the University. Their appointment is made on recommendations of their clinical department faculty through the departmental chairpeople to the Dean of the School of Dental Medicine. To take effect, an appointment or promotion must be reviewed and approved by the School of Dental Medicine's Committee on Faculty Appointments and Promotions and Committee of Professors, utilizing general criteria defined and agreed to by the voting faculty of the school. It must be reviewed and approved in normal course by the Provost's Staff Conference.
>
> Termination of employment for persons who have chosen and entered into work on the non-tenure track is made only because of (1) failure to secure promotion to associate professor by the end of the probationary

period which shall not exceed ten years; (2) attainment of any required retirement age; (3) lack of funds from clinical income to pay their salaries, or (4) for "just cause" as customarily determined within the University.

To assure conformity with nomenclature approved for the University, appointees in the clinical-educator track with a professional rank hold the modified title of Assistant Professor, Associate Professor, or Professor of Clinical Dentistry (or other specialty, as appropriate). That is, a clear and correct modifier is always attached to the professional title.

Initially, there is a three-year appointment for all full-time dental faculty appointed to non-tenured positions. At this time, clinical faculty may choose either a direct appointment to the clinical-educator track, or a seven-year or ten-year tenure track probationary period. In the case of the seven-year probationary track, a decision must be made by the end of the initial three-year appointment to either remain in the seven-year track or to transfer to the ten-year tenure or non-tenure clinical track. Those in the ten-year track must, after six years of service at the latest, choose between the two tracks. No subsequent change from a tenure to a non-tenure track is permitted. Faculty members initially appointed to the clinical-educator track may change to a seven-year traditional tenure track at the completion of the third year of their appointment as a clinical educator. Persons from outside the school faculty with appropriate experience and credentials for initial appointment at senior ranks ordinarily join immediately with the standing Faculty (with tenure) or the Standing Clinical-Educator Faculty (without tenure).

All clinical educators have a written contract with the School of Dental Medicine that contains a clear statement of: the conditions of employment, the circumstances under which the contract can be terminated, the responsibility of the department or other budgetary unit for payment of income and all specific benefits, the right of persons to due process by mechanisms available to all University faculty in the event of grievances of alleged failure to protect the individual rights accorded a faculty member, and the restrictions that all patient care activities will be in facilities under the auspices of the School of Dental Medicine.

Just as the benefits are not restricted to tenured employees of the University, appointees will be entitled to full University faculty benefits. Leaves are not an unconditional benefit, whether for scholarly or other purposes, and are to be granted only when determined on an individual basis to be in the interest of both the individual and the School of Dental Medicine.

A faculty member on this track is required to devote his/her full professional time to activities on behalf of the educational and patient care activities of the School of Dental Medicine. All practice earnings are returned to and managed by the School of Dental Medicine. Salaries conform to School of Dental Medicine policies. The faculty member is subject to University policy on conflict of interest, except that he/she is

not permitted to devote any time to employment in extramural professional practice. Otherwise, persons in this category share all rights and
privileges of other School of Dental Medicine faculty. At no time can
the voting strength of faculty members on the new clinical-faculty track
exceed 30 percent of the voting strength of the Standing Faculty of the
School of Dental Medicine as a whole.

These recommendations are in no way intended to change the status
of or to decrease the rights and obligations of other persons presently on
the full-time faculty of the School of Dental Medicine.[1]

In April 1980 the School of Dental Medicine Faculty Senate approved the
proposal. In June 1981 it was approved by the Board of Trustees of the University. A major obstacle in the path of creating future Model B practices had been
removed.

Other Developments

During the summer of 1980, Dr. Alvin Morris left his position as project director to devote time to a research project on quality assurance, and Deans Cohen
and Cormier became codirectors of the Pennsylvania Experiment. Deborah
Diserens, an educational evaluator, was hired as full-time educational coordinator to oversee the evaluation of the experiment.

YEARS II AND III

The Busch Center

By the beginning of the second year of the experiment, an evaluation team was
selected, the Busch Center of Applied Research, a research and evaluation unit
of the Wharton School of the University of Pennsylvania specializing in the
design and organization of systems. After an initial examination of the Pennsylvania Experiment that included extensive interviews and a questionnaire
given to administrators, faculty members, and students, the Busch Center concluded that before evaluation could occur, a planning and redesign effort was
necessary. Several salient problems were identified, specifically, lack of clarity
among students concerning the objectives of the models, the roles of students
and faculty within the models, and lack of control by students in the operation
of the practices. The center viewed other problems such as ineffective collection practices as reflections of these larger problems; students had little control over and active participation in the practices. Although the original aims
of the experiment were innovative, the existing organization was becoming
increasingly bureaucratic.

In January 1981 the Busch Center reported the results of its systems analysis
to the members of the experiment, identifying the key problems as "lack of
clarity of tasks to be performed" and "lack of control over how the job is being
done [among students]." In February the center proposed an idealized organi-

zational design for the models that became a springboard from which student-faculty teams in each of the models developed their own designs.

Teams of faculty and students within the models met for several months and developed revised organizational structures, emphasizing decentralization and semiautonomous responsibility centers. Student participation in this process was high. A questionnaire administered to students following the planning process revealed a marked change in attitude, emphasizing feelings of greater involvement and control as well as clarity about their roles. Throughout the summer of 1981, the Busch Center aided in the implementation of these new organizational designs.

The Busch Center also began to design an evaluation process during Year II in close collaboration with Dr. Cormier, Ms. Diserens, and several other key faculty participants in the experiment. At an initial meeting in the fall of 1980, it was determined that the evaluation efforts could be organized into three interrelated dimensions: financial, managerial, and educational. It was further agreed that the educational dimension could be defined by measures related to student outcomes in three areas: cognitive, psychomotor, and affective. During Year II, a steering committee composed of traditional and experimental faculty met to identify the measures to be used in the evaluation process. Existing measures (Northeast Regional Boards, grade point average, and so forth) were to be supplemented with several new test instruments to be designed by the appropriate faculty members in collaboration with Ms. Diserens. Thus areas such as human relations skills and work environment could be captured by the evaluation process.

Faculty-Student Issues

By the second year of the experiment, a new set of problems had emerged. It was now clear that the experiment was achieving its objectives—that a school within a school had emerged. Problems with faculty and students outside of the experiment associated with this phenomenon became evident.

Nonexperiment faculty expressed concern about the education of students in Models A and B. Departmental chairpersons, in particular, pointed out that students were graduating from the school without being evaluated by departmental chairpersons (although many departmental faculty members taught part-time in both models, and Drs. Tisot and Casullo could declare a student qualified for graduation in all of the clinical disciplines).

This situation was, of course, a natural outcome of starting a school within a school and of creating a decentralized educational unit. The Pennsylvania Experiment necessitated that control in the school become somewhat decentralized, which naturally created some resistance and concern among dental school faculty.

To address this issue, Dr. Cormier worked with each of the individual departmental chairpersons, developing a specific set of criteria for certifying students for graduation. Students were required to comply with these criteria as well as with those within their respective models. These new requirements were generally minor additions to existing ones, such as one or two rotations into a clinical department in the dental school (or submitting products for review, such as several sets of radiographs). The new standards were implemented in Year II of the experiment. Thus the Pennsylvania Experiment could proceed as an independent system of education, but one that was compliant and closely linked with the traditional dental school departmental structure.

Some resentment on the part of students in the traditional program also emerged in the second year. Some students felt that the students in the experiment were receiving a better education and more attention from the school administration than they were. Attempts were made by the administration to meet the concerns of these students; however, the reality was that a new D.M.D. program had indeed emerged within the school, and comparisons were a natural outcome.

Model G

During the third year of the experiment, a new Model B-type practice, known as Model G, was implemented in a hospital environment (referring to its location at Graduate Hospital in Philadelphia). This practice is still in its developmental stages and is being studied as another model of the faculty-based practice/dental school environment.

The Pennsylvania Experiment officially ended during the summer of 1982. The Busch Center began the aggregation and analysis of its data during this time and submitted its final report on the financial, educational, and managerial results of the experiment in September 1983.

Note

1. Faculty Senate, "University of Pennsylvania Clinician Educator Track for School of Dental Medicine," April 22, 1980.

Evaluation, Part I: Educational Dimension, The Busch Center Report

Chapters 6 and 7 are based on the Busch Center Report on the educational, financial, and managerial dimensions of the Pennsylvania Experiment. Chapter 6 presents the educational data; Chapter 7 presents the financial and managerial data. Some editorial changes have been made; however, the content of these chapters is drawn directly from the Busch Report submitted in 1982 after the completion of the three-year experiment.

Busch Center Report

OVERALL SUMMARY OF EVALUATION

The intent of this evaluation was to be able to communicate to the dental education community the outcomes of the experiment: to say whether it worked successfully or not. The definition of "worked" depends on the group addressed. This evaluation report was addressed to many groups but chose as its language the types of measures most commonly used in dental education. As incomplete as they may be, the standardized and standard-type measures of the mastery of the art and science of dentistry are still the best available for sharing information in a way that can be useful and meaningful to more than a small number of people.

At the same time, it was recognized that the material contained in the report only partially represents the reality which took place during the three years of the experiment. The "clinical impressions" of faculty at the School of Dental Medicine and the growth in the future of the students, for example, are two important sources of data which remain untapped.

A developmental year and two years of data collection allowed for only the beginning of the evaluation of the Pennsylvania Experiment. Follow-up of the classes of students still in school as well as those who have already graduated is essential to understand more fully the impact of the experiment curriculum.

At the time of the evaluation, none of the students in the experiment had gone entirely through the experiment. (The Class of 1983 constituted the first group of students to go entirely through the program, completing their residency in 1984; the evaluation was completed in 1982.) Therefore, the Busch evaluation is presented within the context of these constraints.

Summary of Results

Model B, the dental care center practice, can be characterized as being educationally effective and financially viable. It is perceived by students as a preferable work environment when compared with the traditional program at the School of Dental Medicine. Positive outcomes have not been achieved without considerable problems and growing pains; however, it appears that the Dental Care Center will continue to be a successful model for the education of dentists, if the current level of energy and resources is maintained and improved, and if its unique needs within the university can be accommodated.

Model A, the Paletz Clinic, is educationally effective; however, because Model A is more dependent than Model B on the overall economics of the dental school, it is not likely to be a financially viable model, in its current state, although it can continue to increase productivity with further internal management improvements. It is, like Model B, perceived as a preferable work environment by students when compared with the traditional program. Further, it has demonstrated that a generalist preclinical and clinical curriculum is achieveable and effective.

Of particular significance for the future of the dental profession and dental education are the data regarding service mix and productivity in the two practices. For two years, both the Model A and Model B clinical practices have delivered two to three times the amount of periodontal and preventive and diagnostic services as the national average for general practitioners functioning outside the dental school setting. It appears that these clinical environments are offering students a balanced exposure to the treatment of periodontal disease and dental caries. Model B, which is a private practice environment, appears to facilitate both student and resident productivity. In particular, the productivity data for residents in Model B show promising possibilities for these providers to be significant contributors to revenue for dental schools.

Table 6-1 summarizes the accomplishments of the Pennsylvania Experiment, comparing them to the recommendations of the Long Range Planning Committee.

EDUCATIONAL DIMENSION

The purpose of the evaluation of the educational dimension of the Pennsylvania Experiment was to assure that the curriculum produced outcomes at least

Table 6-1. Implementation of the Recommendations of the Long Range Planning Committee

---

1. That the class size be reduced to eighty students beginning with the class entering in the fall of 1979.

   Implementation
   Entering class reduction to 120 (from 160) students began in September 1982 with additional reductions to 112 in 1983 and 75 students in 1984.

2. That the School of Dental Medicine begin a new curriculum in the fall of 1979, which will include a fifth-year family practice residency program.

   Implementation
   The Pennsylvania Experiment curriculum includes a fifth-year general practice residency. Ten residents participated in 1979–80, twelve in 1981–82, and fourteen in 1982–83 and 1983–84. This program has been accredited as an advanced dental education program in general dentistry and is now in effect.

3. That the preceptorship model of clinical instruction be adopted as the principal method of clinic instruction, and that clinic-based (as exemplified by the current student general group practice) and faculty group practice based preceptorship teams will constitute the normative clinical experiences of the student.

   Implementation
   Eight students and four residents per year received all of their clinical instruction in Model B of the Pennsylvania Experiment, which uses the preceptor model. Forty students and eight residents per year received all of their preclinical and clinical experience in Model A, using a modified preceptorship format.

4. That a system of faculty group practices, under the aegis of the university and staffed by full-time clinical faculty, be instituted.

   Implementation
   The Model B Dental Care Center, a financially self-sustaining group practice, was established during the Pennsylvania Experiment and continues to be successful educationally and financially.

5. That the preclinical technique courses be revised to stress the learning of those basic skills which students will be called upon to apply in the immediate future and to relate the technique course in time to the developing clinical experiences of the student.

   Implementation
   A generalist preclinical sequence was fully implemented in the Pennsylvania Experiment, including earlier clinical exposure through chairside assisting, allowing students to reach clinical readiness sooner. It is now the model for the entire dental school.

6. That the curriculum of the first four years be a balanced experience to broaden the background of the generalist (and reduce the emphasis on the specialties as separate entities).

   Implementation
   An integrated generalist preclinical and clinical program is fully implemented in the Pennsylvania Experiment, including courses and experiences in human behavior, practice management, and teaching skills.

Table 6-1. Implementation of the Recommendations of the Long Range
Planning Committee (continued)

7. That the training of dental specialists be continued, with a cautious eye on the
   changing character of dental practice, and that the consequent need to alter or
   phase out specific specialty training programs be considered as appropriate action
   for the future.

   Implementation

   Specialty training has been continued at the School of Dental Medicine, with a
   reduction in total numbers of students. The primary emphasis of the School of
   Dental Medicine is the training of the generalist.

8. That dental auxiliary education in the school be integrated with the comprehensive
   plan and that dental hygiene education involving basic preparation and possible
   baccalaureate and master's degree programs be developed, and that a study be made
   of the feasibility of increasing the number of dental auxiliary students educated
   with the dental students for efficient team practice.

   Implementation

   Dental hygiene students were trained in the Model A clinical facility; dental
   hygienists and dental hygiene residents were included in the facilities of both Models A and B. Trained dental assistants were also used in Models A and B. Trained
   dental auxiliaries are considered essential in the training of dental students.

9. That mechanisms be implemented concurrently with the new program to ensure
   (a) achievement of the recommendations, (b) adjustments when objectives are not
   achieved, (c) instructional quality, (d) student performance evaluation, and (e) quality of patient care.

   Implementation

   (a) Administrative staff and faculty were in place since September 1979 to implement experimental programs.
   (b) Ongoing review and revision of clinic operations and curriculum took place
   through Pennsylvania Experiment management and evaluation assessments by the
   Busch Center.
   (c) Schoolwide instructor evaluation was implemented.
   (d and e) Student performance and quality of patient care were evaluated through
   students' peer review preclinically and clinically, clinical reviews of student performance, patient satisfaction measures, and coordination of preclinical and clinical evaluation schemes.

10. That, with the reduction in the number of students, a major renovation of the
    Evans Building, plus the necessity of an east court in-fill and/or a faculty practice
    facility, will serve the needs of the school if the above recommendations are ap-
    proved.

    Implementation

    A planning committee is meeting presently to define the size, characteristics,
    and location of a new facility.

comparable academically to those of the ongoing educational program at the School of Dental Medicine. This section describes the results of comparison between three groups of students: Model A, Model B, and Model T (traditional).

Subjects

Three groups of students were compared on a number of educational outcome measures. These groups consist of students from the experimental Models A and B and of students from the traditional curriculum, designated Model T. In some cases, data on an entire class in the Model T curriculum were used for comparisons, and in other cases, data from a randomly sampled control group from Model T were used.

The process of selection and assignment to groups was slightly different for each class. Some students who participated in the experimental curriculum had already completed one, two, and three years of education in the traditional curriculum. Thus increased amounts of information were available about the students and a more extensive screening process could be used, including completion and review of an application asking a student to assess her or his goals for the future and intent to commit to a career in general dentistry, as well as an interview. This process was used in the selection of all members of the experimental group in the Class of 1980 (residents only in Pennsylvania Experiment) the Class of 1981 (senior and residency years in the experiment), and the Class of 1981 (junior, senior, and residency years in the experiment).

Control group students for the classes of 1981 and 1982 were selected by choosing from among the original pool of applicants to the experiment with an effort to match the quintile distribution of students using quintile rank at the time of selection for the experiment.

The classes of 1983, 1984, and 1985 were selected and assigned randomly to experimental and control groups; the experiment was in effect for their entire dental school experiences (all four years). The fact that these groups are more demonstrably "clean" from an experimental point of view is one among many reasons that the data-collection process should be continued in the next few years.

Replacements have been made to both groups at different points in time; these cases are noted in the reports of the individual tests.

Procedures

Anonymity and confidentiality of data were retained through the use of code numbers of all data. All aggregation of data and statistical analyses were completed by the Busch Center staff.

Specific methods and procedures associated with the implementation of each measure are described in sections that report the data.

Measures

The outcome measures used in evaluating the students for both experimental years (1980–81 and 1981–82) are as follows:

1. Students' academic grades
2. National Board examinations
3. Senior treatment planning examination
4. Clinical performance review results (four measures)
5. Northeast Regional Board examinations

The additional measures which were developed or used to assess the educational dimension in 1981–82 are as follows:

1. Patient situation test
2. Patient satisfaction questionnaire
3. Dental hygiene residency questionnaire
4. Junior treatment planning examination
5. Diagnostic radiology examination
6. Student clinical activity (analysis of completed procedures)
7. Junior, senior, and resident service mix profiles
8. Assessment of freshmen and sophomores preclinical skills (six measures)
9. Assessment of mandibular block technique
10. Freshman and sophomore assisted or observed procedures and profile

Constraints

Caveats against overinterpretations of the data presented are offered because compromises were made in the experimental design and samplings. Constraints are always present in research, particularly when the research involves human experimentation. Two constraints are most salient in explaining the limitations on the educational evaluation in this project. First, it would have been preferable to have twenty or thirty students in each of the classes in Model A and in Model B; however, particularly in Model B, the cost would have been prohibitive. As a consequence, differences based on samples of four per class in Model B and eight per class in Model A must be viewed guardedly and must await corroboration over time. If the samples were larger, the measures used here would have been more able to discriminate between groups. Second, in many areas no established instruments were available to fit the needs of the experiment. Therefore, several measures were developed and used only once—during the experimental period. This constraint has not allowed for adequate refinement of the tests or for determination of their reliability or validity. Again, repeated measures over time will help either to corroborate or to disprove the conclusions offered in this report.

In all analyses presented here, Model A and Model B data were compared; if no difference was found, these data were combined for purposes of comparison to Model T data. This procedure served to increase the precision of the comparison of test results. Information on productivity and service data, however, is presented separately.

EDUCATIONAL DATA

Table 6-2 displays the measures used in the educational evaluation, the years in which data were collected, and the educational comparability or difference between Models A/B and T. Also indicated in the table are data that were collected for only Models A and B and not T.

Affective Measures

COMMUNICATION SKILLS

Patient situation test, Classes of 1982, 1983, 1984, 1985, academic year 1981–82.

METHODOLOGY

An important difference between the experimental and traditional curricula is that all experimental students take a human behavior course during the freshman year. The major focus of this course is on interpersonal communication skills and learning to recognize responses that facilitate communication and those that do not.

Based on the work of E. H. Porter[1] and others, Lewis Bernstein and R. Bernstein[2] developed a measure, the patient situation test, which is made up of typical provider-patient incidents, in which a patient's comment to the provider and five possible responses are presented. For each item, the possible responses are "evaluative," "hostile," "probing," "reassuring," and "understanding." The "understanding" response is the choice that best facilitates communication, as demonstrated in research by T. M. Newcomb.[3]

This measure was chosen to determine whether there was any difference between experimental and control students in their ability to recognize "understanding" responses.

The test was administered to experimental and control students in all four classes during the spring of 1982. An assessment of the longevity of the learning can also be derived from the data, since the 1981–82 juniors and seniors took the human behavior course in 1979–80 and the sophomores took it in 1980–81.

Although the ability to recognize "understanding" responses as measured by the test is not the same as using them in patient interviews, the test has been shown to predict actual behavior. In real-life encounters, however, the absolute frequency of understanding responses goes down.[4] Split-half reliabilities for the scales are reported at .74 to .92.

DATA

Experimental and control groups of seniors, juniors, sophomores, and freshmen answered the patient situation test, a seventeen-question test. Their responses were classified into five categories: "evaluative," "hostile," "reassuring," "probing," and "understanding."

Table 6-2. Educational Outcome Measures

Educational Outcome Measures	Year Used		Similar Outcomes in A/B and T	Different Outcomes in A/B and T	Model T Data Not Available
	1980–81	1981–82			
I. Affective:					
1. Patient situation test		x		x	
2. Dental hygiene questionnaire		x		x	
3. Patient satisfaction questionnaire		x	x		
II. Psychomotor (preclinical and clinical):					
4. Preclinical projects (six measures)		x	x		
5. Mandibular block technique		x	x		
6. Chairside assisting profile		x			x
7. Clinical performance reviews (four measures)	x	x	x		
8. Clinical activity analysis		x		x	
9. Northeast Regional Boards	x	x	x		
III. Cognitive:					
10. National board examinations	x	x	x		
11. Grade point averages	x	x	x		
12. Junior treatment planning examination	x	x	x		
13. Senior treatment planning examination		x	x		
14. Diagnostic radiology examination		x	x		

Table 6-3. Patient Situation Test, Class of 1982 (Seniors)

	Control	Experiment	
Evaluative	51	41	
Hostile	27	17	
Reassuring	50	38	
Probing	37	32	
Understanding	22	59	
TOTAL	187	187	$X^2 = 26.3$

Table 6-4. Patient Situation Test, Class of 1983 (Juniors)

	Control	Experiment	
Evaluative	40	30	
Hostile	14	20	
Reassuring	50	32	
Probing	49	35	
Understanding	17	87	
TOTAL	170	204	$X^2 = 20.0$

Seniors (Class of 1982)
Eleven control and eleven experimental students completed the test. The scores for the groups were computed as the number of responses to each of the seventeen questions. Therefore, the total number of responses was $11 \times 17 = 187$ per group.

The distribution of responses for the two groups is seen in Table 6-3.

Juniors (Class of 1983)
Ten control and twelve experimental students completed the test. The distribution of responses to the seventeen questions is seen in Table 6-4.

Sophomores (Class of 1984)
Seven experimental and eleven control students completed the test. The distribution of responses to the seventeen questions is seen in Table 6-5.

Freshmen (Class of 1985)
Twelve experimental and twelve control students completed the test. The distribution of responses to the seventeen questions is seen in Table 6-6.

Table 6-5. Patient Situation Test, Class of 1984 (Sophomores)

	Control	Experiment	
Evaluative	43	23	
Hostile	16	8	
Reassuring	38	25	
Probing	39	24	
Understanding	51	39	
TOTAL	187	119	$X^2 = 7.8$

Table 6-6. Patient Situation Test, Class of 1985 (Freshmen)

	Control	Experiment	
Evaluative	52	22	
Hostile	11	10	
Reassuring	42	38	
Probing	47	34	
Understanding	35	83	
TOTAL	187	187	$X^2 = 20.0$

TESTS PERFORMED

A chi-squared test of homogeneity was performed. For the seniors, juniors, and freshmen the magnitude of the X^2 suggests that the hypothesis that the control and experimental samples were drawn from the same universe is not supported by the data at a $p < .01$ level of significance. In other words, there is a statistically significant difference between the responses of the experimental and control samples for these three classes. Furthermore, most of the discrepancy between the frequencies of the two samples occurs in the "understanding" category. A chi-squared test of homogeneity considering only the remaining four categories shows that for those categories the samples are not significantly different $(p < .01)$. The distribution of responses for the sophomores, however, is not significantly different between the experimental and control groups for any of the dimensions.

CONCLUSION

The senior, junior, and freshman experimental and control students differ significantly regarding the number of "understanding" responses given on the patient situation test, with those in the experiment giving more understanding responses.

DENTAL HYGIENE RESIDENCY SURVEY

METHODOLOGY

A goal of the Pennsylvania Experiment was to develop in students collaborative attitudes and behaviors toward all members of the dental team. Particular emphasis was placed on developing more effective working relations with hygienists. Thus dental students in the experimental program participate in cotherapy of patients with both first- and second-year hygiene students in Model A and licensed hygienists in Model B.

In addition, in July 1981, the first dental hygiene residency program in the country was begun at the School of Dental Medicine. Two 1981 hygiene graduates were chosen for the program. One was assigned to Model A and one to Model B.

Thus students in Models A and B are exposed to hygiene students, residents, and providers as a matter of routine in their clinical practice. In contrast, Model T students participate in cotherapy with hygiene students only, and only on an informal basis, because hygiene students are in a separate bay in the main clinic.

To assess whether there were any differences in attitudes toward hygienists, a questionnaire was designed and developed to measure dental students' attitudes toward hygienists' work and knowledge.[5] To make further comparisons, students from two other dental schools were also sampled: Columbia University and Case Western Reserve. Columbia's dental school has a hygiene program; Case Western does not.

Students from the dental schools of the University of Pennsylvania, Columbia University, and Case Western Reserve University were asked to answer a twelve-item questionnaire, testing attitudes toward dental hygiene procedures (see Appendix VIII). Samples of all years (1982–85) for each school were taken to provide a contrast with the experimental and traditional students. A sample of eleven dental residents in the experimental program of the University of Pennsylvania School of Dental Medicine was also taken and was treated separately.

SAMPLE SIZE

Table 6-7 shows the sample size from each of these groups of respondents to the questionnaire.

RESULTS (TABLE 6-8)

The questionnaire results are presented in Table 6-8 by various groupings. Because of the small sample sizes and the large number of comparisons possible, no statistical tests were performed.

Question 11 shows that a substantial majority of students have no or very limited experience in working with dental hygienists. Their opinions therefore, will reflect their attitudes and judgments based on indirect experience.

Table 6-7. Sample Sizes, Dental Hygiene Residency Survey

Class	Case Western	Columbia	Pennsylvania Experiment Model A and B	Control	Total	Total All Schools
1982	32	18	10	5	15	65
1983	53	7	5	6	11	71
1984	87	5	9	9	18	110
1985	66	7	5	8	13	86
TOTAL	238	37	29	28	57	332

Table 6-8. Responses to Dental Hygiene Residency Survey (percentages)

Question	SD	D	NO	A	SA
1	4.0	8.0	10.5	44.9	37.6
2	4.9	15.3	32.2	34.0	13.5
3	6.3	18.7	21.1	35.3	18.4
4	8.1	15.4	12.7	40.7	23.2
5	12.4	32.7	18.8	26.1	10.0
6	11.4	16.6	22.9	25.3	23.8
7	28.9	37.0	24.4	8.1	1.5
8	22.8	28.5	21.6	23.7	3.3
9	4.5	11.8	24.5	40.0	19.1
10	0.6	2.1	5.7	39.5	52.1

SD = strongly disagree   NO = no opinion
D = disagree   A = agree
    SA = strongly agree

Question 11	
No experience	69.4
Limited experience	17.8
Moderate experience	7.9
Numerous experiences	5.0

There is general agreement that a dental hygienist is a valuable member of a dental practice (Question 10). Consistent with their lack of experience, the respondents have little knowledge about the skills and knowledge of a dental hygienist (Question 5). Also, the respondents believe that hygienists are not as competent as dentists in the areas of emergency procedures and early detection of abnormalities (Questions 7 and 8).

ALL CLASSES SEPARATED BY SCHOOL (TABLE 6-9)

The response patterns of students at all three schools are similar, with a few exceptions. The biggest difference is in the perception of the dental hygienist's ability for early detection of abnormalities (Question 8). Penn dental students (in contrast with the Case and Columbia students) believe that hygienists have that ability. Also, regarding emergency procedures (Question 7) Penn students have a high level of "no opinion" while most of the other students disagree with the statement presented.

Regarding familiarity with the skills and knowledge of the graduate dental hygienist (Question 5), Columbia and Case students seem to differ, while Penn students are evenly divided. This difference might be the result of more exposure of dental students to hygienists' work at Columbia, as reflected in Question 11. With regard to a career, Penn students are relatively more undecided and favor specialization more than the students of the other two schools.

PENN STUDENTS: EXPERIMENTAL AND TRADITIONAL PROGRAMS
(TABLE 6-10)

Penn students of Models A and B are considerably more aware of the skills of dental hygienists than are the students of the traditional program (Question 5). They agree more strongly with the statement that hygienists have similar skills to those of dentists in nonsurgical periodontal therapy (Question 6).

PENN RESIDENTS: EXPERIMENTAL GROUP (TABLE 6-11)

The opinions of this group do not differ significantly from the opinions of other groups with the exception of Question 8 and Question 1. The difference of opinion of this group and of students of both Case Western Reserve and Columbia Universities is very strong. In contrast to students, the residents believe that hygienists are able to detect abnormalities.

Question 3 is not comparable because it pertains to each specific stage of education.

DISCUSSION

It appears that the substantial majority of the students in all the schools sampled have limited or no cotherapy experience with hygienists.

All students sampled agree that the dental hygienist is a valuable member of the dental team. This appears to be a generalized attitude possessed by all dental students given that most of the students sampled here have no experience upon which to base their opinions.

Table 6-9. Responses to Dental Hygiene Residency Survey, All Classes (percentages)

Question	Case Western					Columbia					Pennsylvania				
	SD	D	NO	A	SA	SD	D	NO	A	SA	SD	D	NO	A	SA
1	5.1	8.5	11.1	49.1	26.1	2.7	13.5	2.7	35.1	45.9	0.0	5.6	12.5	32.1	50.0
2	7.0	14.8	36.7	36.5	10.0	0.0	27.0	37.6	21.6	18.9	0.0	10.2	33.9	32.2	23.7
3	5.5	19.9	22.5	33.9	18.2	8.1	13.5	18.9	43.2	16.2	8.6	17.2	17.2	36.2	20.7
4	8.9	14.8	13.9	41.8	20.7	5.4	21.6	2.7	40.5	29.7	6.9	13.8	13.8	36.2	29.3
5	12.7	34.7	20.8	24.2	7.6	8.1	27.0	16.2	35.1	13.5	14.0	28.1	12.3	28.1	17.5
6	13.4	19.7	23.9	25.2	17.6	13.5	13.5	16.2	18.9	37.8	1.8	5.4	23.2	30.4	41.1
7	29.4	39.1	22.3	8.0	1.3	45.9	32.4	21.6	0.0	0.0	15.8	31.6	35.1	14.0	3.5
8	25.6	29.0	23.1	20.2	2.1	21.6	32.6	16.2	27.0	2.7	12.1	24.1	19.0	36.2	8.6
9	4.2	11.4	25.0	40.3	19.1	8.1	13.5	16.2	45.9	16.2	3.5	12.3	28.1	35.1	21.1
10	0.8	2.9	7.6	45.8	42.9	0.0	0.0	2.7	27.0	70.3	0.0	0.0	0.0	21.1	78.9

SD = strongly disagree NO = no opinion
D = disagree A = agree
SA = strongly agree

Question 11	Case	Columbia	Pennsylvania
No experience	77.3	38.3	62.1
Limited experience	15.5	27.7	19.0
Moderate experience	4.2	25.5	8.6
Numerous experiences	2.9	8.5	10.3

Table 6-10. Responses to Dental Hygiene Residency Survey, Penn Students: Experimental and Traditional Programs (percentages)

Question	Experimental					Control				
	SD	D	NO	A	SA	SD	D	NO	A	SA
1	.0	3.4	3.4	27.6	65.3	.0	7.4	22.2	37.0	33.3
2	.0	13.3	16.7	36.7	33.3	.0	6.9	51.7	27.6	13.8
3	10.0	13.3	20.0	36.7	20.0	7.1	21.4	14.3	35.7	21.4
4	9.4	15.6	15.6	21.9	37.5	3.8	11.5	11.5	53.8	19.2
5	3.3	20.0	10.0	36.7	30.0	25.9	37.0	14.8	18.5	3.7
6	3.3	3.3	13.3	36.7	43.3	.0	7.4	33.3	22.2	37.0
7	13.3	36.7	26.7	20.0	3.3	18.5	25.9	44.4	7.4	3.7
8	9.7	32.3	16.1	35.5	6.5	14.8	14.8	22.2	37.0	11.1
9	6.7	10.0	30.0	43.3	10.0	.0	14.8	25.9	25.9	33.3
10	.0	.0	.0	10.0	90.0	.0	.0	.0	33.3	66.7

SD = strongly disagree   NO = no opinion
D = disagree   A = agree
  SA = strongly agree

Question 11	Experimental	Control
No experience	56.7	67.9
Limited experience	23.3	14.3
Moderate experience	6.7	10.7
Numerous experiences	13.3	7.1

Table 6-11. Responses to Dental Hygiene Residency Survey, Penn Residents, Experimental Group (percentages)

Question	SD	D	NO	A	SA
1	0.0	0.0	0.0	18.2	81.8
2	0.0	9.1	18.2	45.5	27.3
3	10.0	20.0	40.0	20.0	10.0
4	0.0	18.2	18.2	54.5	9.1
5	0.0	18.2	18.2	45.5	18.2
6	9.1	9.1	18.2	18.2	45.5
7	63.6	18.2	18.2	0.0	0.0
8	0.0	36.4	9.1	45.5	9.1
9	9.1	27.3	9.1	45.5	9.1
10	0.0	0.0	0.0	9.1	90.9

SD = strongly disagree   NO = no opinion
D = disagree   A = agree
     SA = strongly agree

Question 11

No experience	18.2
Limited experience	18.2
Moderate experience	27.3
Numerous experiences	36.4

Question 12

Private practice	72.7
Established dental clinic/practice	9.1
Specialization	0.0
Uncertain	18.2
Other	0.0

Most respondents feel that hygienists are not as competent as dentists in the areas of emergency procedures, early detection of abnormalities, and nonsurgical periondontal therapy. Penn dental students, in particular the residents in the experimental program, as contrasted with Case and Columbia students, believe that hygienists can detect abnormalities. Regarding the hygienist's capability to do emergency procedures, Penn students have a high level of no opinion while the other students disagree. Penn students of Models A and B agree more strongly that hygienists have similar skills to those of dentists in nonsurgical periodontal therapy than do other students. Also, students with clinical experience assess hygienists' emergency skills more positively.

In summary, these data suggest that the additional exposure to the expanding role of the dental hygienist created in the experiment produces a more positive assessment of hygienists' skills. The data need further confirmation with larger samples.

PATIENT SATISFACTION QUESTIONNAIRE

METHODOLOGY
Patients who were being treated in Models A, B, and T were asked to complete a questionnaire evaluating their dentists and the services provided by the clinic.[6] Patient satisfaction questionnaires were distributed by the receptionist in each of the clinical areas to patients while they were waiting to be seen. New patients were not sampled.

The questionnaire consisted of nineteen questions that measure the following four dimensions of the patients' satisfaction: dentist's personality (P), dentist's technical ability (T), office relations (O), and financial relations (F). Every question consisted of a statement for which the patient marked a number in a scale from 1 to 5, 1 meaning strong disagreement and 5 meaning strong agreement.

The patients' answers were organized by clinic (A, B, and T) and by the dental student's class (junior or senior).

DATA
For each group an average level of satisfaction was computed for all four dimensions. The results are presented in Table 6-12. The level of satisfaction was calculated as the percentage of maximum satisfaction (total agreement with positive statements and strong disagreement with statements formulated in a negative way). For example, for Model A, juniors received an average score of 94.1 percent on the personality dimension, with 100 percent representing "maximum satisfaction."

RESULTS AND CONCLUSIONS
No statistically significant differences were found. This result is most interesting in that the patients were as satisfied with seniors as they were with

Table 6-12. Level of Patients' Satisfaction, Models A, B, and T*

	Model A	Model B	Model T
Juniors:			
P	N = 7 (94.1%)	N = 5 (89.2%)	N = 28 (91.7%)
T	N = 7 (92.7%)	N = 5 (90.0%)	N = 29 (85.5%)
O	N = 7 (91.1%)	N = 5 (87.5%)	N = 27 (83.0%)
F	N = 7 (95.5%)	N = 5 (92.5%)	N = 27 (83.3%)
Seniors:			
P	N = 11 (90.9%)	N = 8 (91.7%)	N = 18 (94.4%)
T	N = 10 (83.0%)	N = 7 (87.1%)	N = 18 (88.3%)
O	N = 9 (86.1%)	N = 6 (84.4%)	N = 15 (87.1%)
F	N = 10 (84.4%)	N = 7 (87.5%)	N = 18 (86.1%)

*The letters, P, T, O, and F represent the four dimensions of personality, technical ability, office relations, and financial relations.

juniors. In addition, no differences were found in satisfaction of treatment among the three settings. These data are based on small sample sizes; therefore, it is recommended that additional samples be obtained in the future.

Psychomotor Measures

ASSESSMENT OF FRESHMEN AND SOPHOMORES PRECLINICAL SKILLS, 1981–82 ACADEMIC YEAR

METHODOLOGY

It was hypothesized that the integration of disciplines into one preclinical curricular track (referred to as general dentistry) taught by generalist educators would bring students to a level of mastery of preclinical skills equal to that of the students in the traditional curriculum.

A steering committee of faculty, who planned the design for the evaluation of the clinical and preclinical educational dimensions of the experiment, selected the following six preclinical products as indicators of the level of students' preclinical psychomotor development:

Freshmen (Class of 1985)
Molar waxing (#3)
Cl. II Amalgam preparation (#29 MO)
Cl. I Amalgam preparation (#30 O)
Cl. III DFG preparation

Sophomores (Class of 1984)
Full upper and lower denture setup
Three-unit provisional bridge

All of the preclinical projects were produced by the students in both the experimental and the control groups as practical examinations during their respective laboratory courses. One faculty member from each curriculum (experimental and control) participated in a blind review of all twenty-four practicals. Names and identifying marks were removed from products, and each product was given a code number.

Each rater assessed each product, using a previously agreed-upon set of criteria and rating scale. When each rater had finished his or her individual ratings, the two raters reconciled any differences in their ratings and reported the reconciled score as well.

RESULTS
For each of the measures, the differences between the control and experimental groups were not statistically significant ($p < .01$). The data for each of the six procedures are presented in detail here.

MOLAR WAXING PRACTICAL: TOOTH #3, CLASS OF 1985

DATA
The control and experimental students' products were graded by two instructors, and a reconciled score was recorded using the following scale:

0 = Failure: Unacceptable; both concept and technique missing
1–3 = C: Missing some concepts, but demonstrating some under-
               standing
4–6 = B: Concepts correct with errors in waxing
7–9 = A: Concepts correct; neat; minor to no errors in waxing

In rendering a score the following criteria were considered: (1) landmark relations, (2) contours, (3) contact points, (4) outline forms, (5) occlusal anatomy, and (6) neatness and definition.

No ratings differed by more than one numeric grade. Further, the reconciled grade arrived at by the two raters was always one of the previously rendered scores. Therefore, rater reliability was assumed. Using the reconciled score, the statistics for the control and the experimental groups are as shown in Table 6-13.

Table 6-13. Molar Working Practical, Tooth #3, Class of 1985

	Control	Experiment
N	12.00	12.00
Mean	3.58	3.25
St. dev.	2.46	2.25

Table 6-14. Operative Preclinical Practicals, Class of 1985

	C1 II Amalgam		C1 III DFG		C1 I Amalgam	
	Experiment	Control	Experiment	Control	Experiment	Control
Sample size	12	12	12	12	12	12
Mean	3.67	3.75	4.50	4.00	2.42	3.75
St. dev.	1.436	1.765	1.679	2.796	2.065	1.483

CLASS OF 1985, OPERATIVE PRECLINICAL PRACTICALS: #29MO C1 II AMALGAM PREP; LOWER C1 III DFG PREP; #300 C1 I AMALGAM PREP

DATA

Twelve experimental and twelve control students performed three clinical tasks that were rated by two raters using the following scale:

    0: Unacceptable concept or skill level
    1–3: Serious errors in concept or skill, but clinically acceptable
    4–6: Some errors in concept or skill, but generally good performance
    7–9: Minor errors in skill only, but very good to excellent performance

The raters reconciled their scores and reported this grade as well as their individual ratings. Of the individual scores given by each rater for each procedure, no score was more than one unit from the other score. Therefore, rater reliability was assumed.

The statistics for each procedure using the reconciled scores are shown in Table 6-14.

FULL DENTURE SETUP PRACTICAL, CLASS OF 1984

DATA

Students were rated by two raters using four categories; A, B, C, or fail. The following are the numerical values and criteria associated with each rating:

    A = 1: (a) Correct antero-posterior and mesiolingual inclination and position of upper and lower anterior teeth
          (b) Correct buccolingual position of upper and lower arch, plane of occlusion, and light centric occlusion
          (c) No wax on occlusal surfaces and clean setup
    B = 2: Minor discrepancies in one of the above categories
    C = 3: Major discrepancies in one of the above categories
    I = 4: Major discrepancies in two or more of the above categories.

The grades of the two raters were reconciled and are summarized in Table 6-15.

Table 6-15. Full Denture Setup Practical,
Class of 1984

	Experiment	Control
N	13	12
Mean	2.231	2.667
St. dev.	0.832	0.778

Table 6-16. Three-Unit Provisional Bridge
Practical, Class of 1984

	Experiment	Control
N	12	12
Mean	2.22	2.60
St. dev.	0.476	0.629

THREE UNIT PROVISIONAL BRIDGE PRACTICAL, CLASS OF 1984

DATA
Students were graded by two raters, using a scale of 0 to 4. The grades of both raters were reconciled and are summarized in Table 6-16.

**CLINICAL EVALUATION OF MANDIBULAR BLOCK TECHNIQUE,
SPRING 1982**

METHODOLOGY
The rationale for administering a clinical evaluation of local anesthetic technique, specifically the administration of a mandibular block, was to determine whether there is a significant difference between the performance levels of the Pennsylvania Experiment students and the traditional curriculum students as a result of a difference in preclinical teaching hours, in a controlled laboratory setting of fourteen hours for the Pennsylvania Experiment students as compared to three hours for traditional students.

The clinical evaluation was directed at the twelve third-year Pennsylvania Experiment students and a matching number of traditional students. (Three control group students, however, did not show up for the evaluation.) The students were matched with a partner from the other group. There were two test administration dates.

In order to improve reliability, the three evaluators observed each student's injection simultaneously and then independently scored the performance. This process was used for all twenty-one students. Each observation took approximately fifteen minutes.

DATA

Each student performing a mandibular block injection was evaluated on fifteen aspects of injection technique by three raters. The scoring choices for each aspect were as follows:

0 = student did not perform task
1 = task performed but the student needs improvement
2 = task performed acceptably

For each student, the average of the total scores given by the three raters was computed. For the "raw" scores, discrepancies which one rater scored a 1 or 2 were eliminated from the analysis. The total scores were then factored-up accordingly so that all total scores were comparable. For example, if two dimensions were eliminated and the total score of the remaining 13 dimensions was 19, the total score, 19, would be multiplied by 15/13 and reported as 22.

Out of the 315 classifications, 17 or 5.4 percent were eliminated because of such discrepancies. There did not seem to be a pattern to the areas eliminated. Of the remaining classifications, 60 percent were in total agreement.

The statistics for the control and experimental groups are given in Table 6-17.

TEST PERFORMED AND RESULTS

A variance-corrected t-test for mean equality indicates that the population means are not significantly different at an alpha level of significance of $p < .01$ or less.

CONCLUSION

There is no evidence that the experimental students' performance on mandibular block technique differs from that of the control group.

Table 6-17. Mandibular Block Technique

	Experiment	Control
N	12	9
Mean	25.7	24.2
St. dev.	1.3	3.3

NUMBER AND PERCENTAGE OF PROCEDURES FOR WHICH FRESHMAN AND SOPHOMORE STUDENTS ASSISTED OR OBSERVED (SEPTEMBER 1981–APRIL 1982, CLASSES OF 1984 AND 1985)

METHODOLOGY
One innovation of the experiment curriculum which was considered important was the addition of the chairside assisting course for freshmen and sophomores. Throughout the year, students in these two groups were asked to record the procedure(s) for which they assisted or which they observed in their weekly clinical sessions in order that the distribution of student preclinical exposure to clinical service could be described.

DATA
Table 6-18 presents the data for the 1981–82 academic year.

TESTS PERFORMED AND CONCLUSION
Based upon a chi-square test for homogeneity, there is no significant difference $(p < .01)$ between the distribution of procedures assisted or observed by the sophomore and freshman experimental students.

CLINICAL PERFORMANCE REVIEWS: CLASSES OF 1982 AND 1983, 1981–82 ACADEMIC YEAR

The following sections present the comparison of the pass/fail rates of the control and experimental students in the Class of 1982 and the Class of 1983 on the clinical performance reviews (CPRs), taken during the 1981–82 academic year. The following CPRs were taken:

Seniors (Class of 1982)	*Juniors (Class of 1983)*
Direct filling gold	Amalgam
Complete denture	Composite resin

RESULTS
As with the preclinical measures, no statistically significant differences were seen between experiment and control students $(p < .01)$.

STUDENTS' CLINICAL ACTIVITY, ANALYSIS OF COMPLETED PROCEDURES, JULY 1981–JUNE 1982

DATA
The clinical activity of both juniors and seniors in Models A, B, and T was registered for the period from July 1981 to June 1982. The mean and standard deviations of the number of times a specific procedure was performed were computed for several procedures. The data are presented in Tables 6-19 and 6-20.

Table 6-18. Chairside Assisting, Classes of 1984 and 1985

	Perio	OP	RE	FP	RP	OM	OS	EN	OR	MI	PR	Total
Sophomores	74	232	41	18	13	15	20	40	11	4	0	468
(Class of 1984)	16%	50%	9%	4%	3%	3%	4%	9%	2%	–		
Freshmen	42	106	32	8	4	1	13	16	1	1	0	224
(Class of 1985)	19%	47%	14%	4%	2%	–	6%	7%	–	–		

Perio = periodontics   OP = restorative without lab
RE = restorative with lab   FP = fixed prosthetics
RP = removable prosthetics   OM = oral medicine
OS = oral surgery procedures   EN = endodontic procedures
OR = orthodontics   MI = other procedures
PR = preventive

Table 6-19. Quantity of Work Produced, Class of 1983 (Juniors)

Procedure	Model A (N = 8)		Model B (N = 4)		Model T (N = 138)	
	Mean	St. Dev.	Mean	St. Dev.	Mean	St. Dev.
Endodontics:	5.87	3.4821	5.75	2.9861	3.6014	2.1016
Restorative:						
Amalgams	40.87	14.8173	36.00	12.7802	41.355	16.3197
Resins	23.5	12.4442	24.25	5.909	14.8695	8.8597
DFG's	1.87	1.126	2.25	2.2174	3.0869	2.7985
Inlay/onlay	.25	.4629	1.0	2.0	.8405	1.2571
Single crowns	1.0	1.6036	3.0	3.4641	1.3695	1.8486
Bridges	1.37	3.1139	2.0	2.4495	.2318	.7075
Removable (partial)	.37	.5176	3.0	3.559	.3043	.731
Removable (complete)	.25	.7072	1.75	1.2583	.3695	.8885
Periodontics:						
Scaling	7.87	6.2436	11.5	7.5498	10.2753	3.4148
Appliances	.62	.744	1.25	1.2583	.8333	1.1307
Surgery	2.12	1.126	2.25	1.5	2.3913	1.9869
Oral surgery:						
Extractions	9.5	5.8064	10.75	6.9462	9.9057	4.9874

Table 6-20. Quantity of Work Produced, Class of 1982 (Seniors)

Procedure	Model A (N = 7)		Model B (N = 4)		Model T (N = 135)	
	Mean	St. Dev.	Mean	St. Dev.	Mean	St. Dev.
Endodontics:	6.00	1.9149	11.00	3.6515	3.3555	1.6949
Restorative:						
Amalgams	42.00	16.563	49.25	19.5683	31.1629	11.4951
Resins	26.7142	11.5861	22.5	5.9161	10.40	5.6081
DFG's	2.1428	.69	4.00	4.3205	3.6888	2.7221
Inlay/onlay	1.7142	.9512	3.25	2.63	1.4	1.192
Single crowns	5.8571	3.0783	9.0	6.0	4.9629	3.0771
Bridges	6.2857	4.6085	6.0	2.4495	1.8296	1.1365
Removable (partial)	4.8571	1.8645	6.0	2.708	2.074	1.2436
Removable (complete)	6.1428	1.8644	4.0	1.8258	3.5333	1.6653
Periodontics:						
Scaling	3.1428	2.5448	19.5	14.5258	4.2	2.3462
Appliances	1.0	.8165	2.5	1.7321	.9037	1.0641
Surgery	3.425	2.9921	3.75	1.7078	2.7185	2.0061
Oral surgery:						
Extractions	13.4285	5.8554	15.25	13.7204	13.9555	6.2257

The sizes of the samples are very different. The accuracy of the estimates of the mean values is much higher for Model T than for Models A or B. Almost 50 percent of all possible comparisons between A and T, and B and T for juniors and seniors cannot be performed with the usual t-test for equality of means because the samples present significantly different standard deviations. Further investigation with increased sample sizes should take place to enable more reliable conclusions to be made on procedure-by-procedure comparison. Overall activity in A, B, and T was compared using a nonparametric test.

ANALYSIS OF COMPLETED PROCEDURES

a) Comparison of Model A and Model B

Analyzing the results for juniors and seniors of these two groups yields no significant differences ($p < .01$). Procedures such as inlay/onlay, single crowns, and partial removable dentures for juniors; and DFG, inlay/onlay, scaling, appliances, and extractions for seniors deserve further investigation because the two groups present significantly different variances.

b) Comparison of Models A and B with Model T

For juniors, there are significant differences in only two categories of procedures ($p < .01$).

Among seniors, the number of categories containing significant differences is greater, suggesting that the difference of the level of activity between students in the experimental programs and in the traditional program increases in the senior year.

c) Comparisons of overall activity

To compare the total number of procedures completed in each model, nonparametric signed tests were performed on the means of all thirteen procedure areas. The tests suggest that the overall level of activity of Models A and T is similar and that the level of Model B is significantly higher than those of Models A or T ($p < .01$).

CONCLUSION

It appears that there is more clinical activity, as measured by completed procedures, in Model B than in both A and T and that Model A students have a tendency to complete more work than T students (although the difference is not significant). Further, the difference in activity level appears to be accentuated in the senior year. These differences occurred even though Model T students have 4 days per week of chair time available, whereas Models A and B students have approximately two and one-half days per week, indicating significant differences between students in the experimental and traditional curricula in the area of clinical activity.

NORTHEAST REGIONAL BOARD EXAMS, SPRING 1982, CLASS OF 1982

METHODOLOGY

The Northeast Regional Board Examination is the licensure exam given to graduating seniors who wish to practice dentistry in the northeastern part of the United States.

Students in the experimental and control groups took the Northeast Regional Board exams in May 1982. The following are the data and comparisons of each subscale of the exam.

DATA

Students are tested on a scale from 0 to 100 in five areas: comprehensive treatment planning (CTP); diagnosis, oral medicine, and radiology (DOR); restorative (RES); prosthetics (PROS); and periodontics (PERI). The grades of the experimental group (n = 11) and of the control group (n = 12) were recorded and are summarized in Table 6-21.

In the control group, there was one outlier observation in the areas of restorative and periodontics which increased the standard deviation of the scores for these areas. Therefore, calculations were made first including these outlier observations (Table 6-21) and then excluding them (Table 6-22).

TESTS PERFORMED

A t-test for equality of means was performed for the areas of CTP, DOR, and PROS. Based upon this test, the hypothesis of equal means between the exper-

Table 6-21. Northeast Regional Board Examinations, Class of 1982

	CTP	DOR	RES	PROS	PERI
Experiment:					
Mean	86.45	85.55	85.09	88.36	87.00
St. dev.	5.165	4.613	4.763	4.178	3.975
Control:					
Mean	86.58	87.25	81.00	85.33	84.00
St. dev.	5.035	4.957	12.548	5.549	13.239

Table 6-22. Northeast Regional Board Examinations, Class of 1982

	RES	PERI
Mean	84.36	87.64
St. dev.	4.884	4.273

imental and control groups for the CTP, DOR, and PROS cannot be rejected ($p < .01$). For the RES and PERI areas, the Kruskal-Wallis test indicated that the hypothesis of equal means cannot be rejected ($p < .01$).

CONCLUSION

The performance of the control and experimental students on the Northeast Regional Board Examination was not significantly different.

Cognitive Measures

CLASS OF 1982, THE 1982 NATIONAL BOARD EXAMINATION: PART II, 1981– 1982 ACADEMIC YEAR

METHODOLOGY

The National Board Examination is given to graduating seniors in the December before their graduation. It is a didactic prerequisite for licensure in the United States given to all dental students in accredited dental schools. There are two parts: Part I tests basic science concepts in dental anatomy, microbiology, physiology, biochemistry, gross human anatomy, pathology, and neuroanatomy, and is given at the end of the second year of dental school. Part II tests clinical science concepts in operative dentistry, oral pathology, radiology, endodontics, and periodontics and is given in December of the senior year of dental school. Part II for the Class of 1982 is reported below.

DATA

The students are evaluated by the National Board examiners in seven areas. The statistics for the experimental and control groups are reported in Table 6-23.

TESTS PERFORMED AND RESULTS

A t-test for mean equality indicated that the control and experimental students do not differ significantly on any of the seven dimensions measured by the National Board Examination ($p < .01$). These results differ from the 1982 National Board Examination results, in which a significant difference occurred for the ENDO/PERIO dimension, with the control group scoring higher than the experimental group.

CONCLUSION

The performance of the control and experimental students is not significantly different for any of the seven areas measured by the National Board Examination.

Table 6-23. National Board Examination, Part II, Class of 1982

	Oper. Den.	Pharm.	Prost. Den.	Os. Anes.	Ortho. Pedo.	Oral Path. Perio.	Endo. Perio.	Avg.
Control: N = 12								
Mean	86.6	85.0	86.1	89.6	86.6	87.6	90.3	87.3
St. dev.	5.8	4.5	4.2	4.6	5.9	6.0	4.8	4.3
Experiment: N = 9								
Mean	91.1	86.3	89.2	87.7	81.0	87.8	91.1	88.8
St. dev.	6.2	6.3	6.6	7.0	5.3	6.5	4.3	5.3

GRADES FOR ACADEMIC YEAR 1981–1982, CLASSES OF 1985, 1984, 1983, AND 1982

METHODOLOGY

Throughout the four years of the curriculum there were some courses which experimental and control students took together and some which they took separately. To assess the relative work loads of the noncommon aspects of the curriculum, and any effects they might have on academic performance, a comparison was made of students' grade point averages (GPA) in jointly taken courses.

The courses included in the calculation of this partial GPA for each class are listed below.

The data are presented in the following sections by class.

Freshmen: Class of 1985: Biochemistry, Histology, Embryology and Genetics; Morphodynamics of the Human Body; Growth and Development and Cephalometrics; Radiologic Anatomy; Neuroanatomy; Anatomy Dissection; Physiology-Pharmacology; Form and Function of the Masticatory System; Restorative Dentistry; Orthodontics/Pedodontics I; Radiology; Dental Care Systems.

Sophomores: Class of 1984: General and Oral Pathology; Microbiology; Clinical Pharmacology; Orthodontics/Pedodontics II; Oral Medicine; Anesthesia and Pain Control; Diagnostic Radiology.

Juniors: Class of 1983: Form and Function of the Masticatory System; Restorative Dentistry; Pediatric Dentistry; Preclinical Periodontics; TEAM; Preventive and Interceptive Orthodontics Clinic.

Seniors: Class of 1982: Orthodontics/Pedodontics Dentistry; Hospital Extramural Assignment.

ANALYSIS

A weighted average was computed for each student using the credit hours of the courses as relative weights and assigning the following numbers to the alphabetic grades: A = 3, B = 2, C = 1, Failure = 0. Incompletes were not considered. The overall average of each group was computed. The statistics for each group are shown in Tables 6-24–6-27.

Table 6-24. Grades for Academic Years 1981–1982, Class of 1985

	Experiment	Control
N	12	12
Mean	2.01	1.92
St. dev.	0.28	0.43

Table 6-25. Grades for Academic Years 1981–1982, Class of 1984

	Experiment	Control
N	13	12
Mean	1.826	1.809
St. dev.	0.504	0.431

Table 6-26. Grades for Academic Year 1981–1982, Class of 1983

	Experiment	Control
N	12	12
Mean	2.077	1.836
St. dev.	0.277	0.378

Table 6-27. Grades for Academic Year 1981–1982, Class of 1982

	Experiment	Control
N	11	12
Mean	1.96	2.05
St. dev.	0.45	0.36

TESTS PERFORMED

A t-test for equality of means indicates that the two groups do not differ significantly ($p < .01$).

CONCLUSION

The grade point averages of the control and experimental students in all four classes for the courses taken in common were not significantly different. The same result was obtained for the four classes for the academic year 1980–81.

TREATMENT PLANNING, CLASSES OF 1983 AND 1984

The steering committee for the evaluation of the preclinical and clinical aspects of the experiment determined that, since integration of disciplines was a major thrust of the experimental curriculum, the degree to which this integration was reflected in student skills should be measured. Therefore, the treatment planning skills of both junior and senior students were assessed. To this end, two examinations were developed; the construction of each is discussed below.

JUNIOR TREATMENT PLANNING EXAMINATION

One clinical faculty member from the traditional program and one from the experimental program were asked to develop and administer an examination that would assess the juniors' basic treatment planning skills (i.e., treatment selection, treatment sequencing, simple diagnosis).

An eighteen-item short-answer test was developed in which students were presented in each item with a brief patient history and chief complaint (see Appendix IX). For each patient situation, students were asked to do the following:

(1) Select the treatment(s) they would perform from a preestablished list of treatments on the first page of the exam.
(2) Write these treatments in the sequence in which they should be done.
(3) Indicate the tooth or area of the mouth that would be treated at each step.

DATA

Students were graded by two raters, who used a scale from 0 to 72 with a possible range of 0 to 4 for each question. The grades were averaged, and the statistics for these groups are seen in Table 6-28.

TESTS PERFORMED

A t-test for equality of means indicated that the hypothesis that the mean for both the experimental and control groups are equal cannot be rejected $(p < .01)$.

CONCLUSION

Because the examination had never been administered before, the results should be considered as a pretest. Given the pretest nature, no inference re-

Table 6-28. Treatment Planning Examination, Class of 1983

	Experiment	Control
N	12	10
Mean	60.958	63.9
St. dev.	4.240	3.221

garding the results is warranted. The recommendation is that based upon what was learned, the examination be further refined and be administered again.

SENIOR TREATMENT PLANNING EXAMINATION

A more complex examination was required to assess the skills of graduating seniors.

After a comprehensive national search for an established measure, it was determined that no currently available instrument would satisfy the needs of this project. Three faculty members, one from the experiment and two from the traditional program, developed such a measure.

A pilot form of the instrument was developed and tested in May 1981. Feedback from students on this test yielded recommendations for revisions that were incorporated into the test development effort in 1981–82. An intensive effort was then undertaken beginning in September 1981 to refine the measure further. The test that resulted was composed of four parts all relating to a single case:

Part IA: Students were asked to list the diagnosis and corresponding etiology for the case.

Part IB: Students were asked to list the sequence of treatment they would perform, noting specific procedures and teeth or areas.

Part II: Students were asked to indicate on a grid the diagnosis and treatment for each tooth.

Part III: This section consisted of thirty multiple-choice items about the case.

Part IV: This section asked questions that would help the authors in grading the students' work:
1. Students were asked if they would now change anything in Sections I or II after having completed Section III.
2. Students were asked if they would refer all or part of the treatment in the case.

A copy of the examination is included in Appendix X. Students were also given thirteen color photographs of the case, a case history, a periodontal charting, and a black and white print of the full-mouth series of X-rays for the case. The test was administered at the end of April 1982. No time limit was placed on the test. All students were required to hand in each section of the test before completing the subsequent section.

COMPREHENSIVE TREATMENT PLANNING EXAMINATION: PARTS IA AND IB SENIORS, CLASS OF 1982

DATA

Students answered two questions in Part IA, identified here as diagnosis and etiology, and one question in Part IB.

Table 6-29. Scoring System for Treatment Planning
Examination

A	A−	B+	B	B−	C+	C	C−	F
10	9	8	7	6	5	4	3	0

Table 6-30. Treatment Planning Examination, Class of 1982

	Diagnosis		Etiology		Treatment Plan	
	Experiment	Control	Experiment	Control	Experiment	Control
N	11	11	11	11	11	9
Mean	4.576	5.758	3.970	4.848	5.788	4.939
St. dev.	2.721	3.270	3.057	3.045	1.922	3.105

The answers were classified by three different raters using a scale from A to
C-minus and F for an unacceptable answer.

The scores of the eleven experimental students and of the eleven control
students were translated into a numerical scale as shown in Table 6-29.

All the sixty-six classifications of each rater were compared to the correspon-
dent score of the other raters. Only 5 percent differed by one category and none
differed by more than two categories. Therefore, rater reliability was assumed.

For each student, the scores of the three raters were assumed and averaged.

The statistics for the control and experimental groups by examination part
are shown in Table 6-30.

TESTS PERFORMED

A t-test for equality of means indicates that there are no significant differences
in the responses of the two groups for any of the sections ($p < .01$).

Two students in the control group failed to answer all questions.

A t-test for equality of means was performed without considering the students in both samples who failed to answer two or more questions.

The results are still not significantly different ($p < .01$) (see Table 6-31).

CONCLUSION

Given the pretest nature, no inference regarding the results is warranted. The
recommendation is that based upon what was learned, the examination be further refined and administered again next year.

Table 6-31. Treatment Planning Examination, Class of 1982

| | Diagnosis | | Etiology | | Part IB | |
	Experiment	Control	Experiment	Control	Experiment	Control
N	9	9	9	9	9	9
Mean	5.59	7.04	4.85	5.89	6.00	6.04
St. dev.	1.69	1.80	2.62	2.21	2.04	2.14

Table 6-32. Treatment Planning Examination, Part III, Class of 1982

	Experiment	Control
Sample Size	11	11
Mean	40.82	39.82
St. dev.	5.67	7.11

COMPREHENSIVE EXAMINATION, PART III, SENIORS, CLASS OF 1982

DATA
Students answered thirty multiple choice questions with scores of 0, 1, or 2. The maximum score of Part III of the test is 60 (see Table 6-32).

TESTS PERFORMED
A t-test for equality of means indicates that the sample means do not differ significantly at a $p < .01$ level of significance.

CONCLUSION
Because of the pretest nature of the results, no conclusion is warranted.

DIAGNOSTIC RADIOLOGY, CONTROL AND EXPERIMENTAL GROUPS, SPRING 1982

METHODOLOGY
The intent of this examination was to test the students' diagnostic ability in localized dental and systemic medical and dental pathogenesis likely to be encountered in general practice. Technique slides were included in an effort to evaluate the students' knowledge of technique and processing without having to take radiographs. Slides testing the diagnosis of caries and periodontal

disease were also included. In addition, there was a section devoted to radiology law.

The examination was given to seniors as late in the fourth year as possible so that their radiology experience would be as broad as possible. (Also, the radiology pathology courses do not conclude until the end of the third year so it is possible that juniors would not have encountered some of the pathologic conditions clinically or didactically.) There were two test administration dates. A total of eleven experimental and eleven control group students took the exam.

A faculty member from the traditional program was present during the examination to answer questions for both the control and experimental groups at the same time. Both groups' examinations were coded so that grading was unbiased.

DATA

Each student was evaluated on the following areas: (1) pathology/anatomy; (2) technique/processing; (3) radiology law, and (4) caries/periodontics. The total score for each student was computed. For all areas the lowest score is the best. The maximum scores (worst) for each area are 64, 36, 20, and 16 respectively.

The statistics for the experimental and control groups are shown in Table 6-33.

TESTS PERFORMED AND RESULTS

Individuals in the experimental group performed consistently better on all areas, i.e., had lower scores, than those in the control group. Using a t-test, however, none of the differences were significant at $p < .01$.

CONCLUSION

There is no evidence that the experiment students' performance on the diagnostic radiology examination differs significantly from the performance of the control students.

Table 6-33. Diagnostic Radiology Test

	Experiment (N = 11)					Control (N = 11)				
	1	2	3	4	Total	1	2	3	4	Total
Mean	23.1	16.5	5.3	3.1	47.9	25.7	17.8	5.5	3.6	52.6
St. dev.	8.0	4.6	2.1	2.2	10.4	10.2	5.9	2.7	1.7	13.0
(Mean/max Score × 100)	36.1	45.7	26.4	19.3		40.2	49.5	27.3	22.2	

Overall Discussion of Educational Results

These results demonstrate that according to conventional educational measures the Pennsylvania Experiment curriculum results in students attaining a level of achievement equivalent to that of traditional students in preclinical and clinical cognitive and psychomotor skills. Further, this comparability of educational outcome is achieved using generalist educators, in an integrated, restructured, and accelerated general dentistry preclinical and clinical curriculum, which allows for inclusion of additional undergraduate educational experiences. These include: (1) earlier and extended clinical experiences made possible by dental assisting and an accelerated preclinical curriculum, (2) a human behavior course, and (3) collaborative cotherapy with dental hygiene students and hygiene residents. The results hold true for students in Model A and in Model B, in which faculty have responsibility for both education and income generation. The data also reveal that these additional educational experiences result in measurable differences in outcomes when Model A and Model B students are compared with other students.

The increased emphasis on the preservation of the natural dentition through delivery of preventive periodontal services to the patients appears to have been realized. When the service mix profiles of residents, seniors, and juniors in Models A and B are compared with national averages of general practice service mix, as reported by C. W. Douglass and J. M. Day,[7] there are striking differences in oral diagnosis and prevention and in peridontics. In both these areas, there is almost twice the percent of effort in the experiment programs as in the traditional program.

Earlier and extended clinical experience made possible by clinical dental assisting by dental students and an accelerated preclinical curriculum appear to result in junior and senior students in Models A and B completing more procedures overall than Model T students. Moreover, this is achieved within the context of two and one-half days per week of available chair time, as compared to four days a week in Model T.

The human behavior course has had a positive effect on the attitudes of experiment students, as manifested by the results of the patient situation test, a measure of interpersonal communication style. Experimental students selected more "understanding" responses than did traditional students. These data reinforce the premise that an explicit curriculum in behavioral science can develop specific communication skills which do not disappear over time.

Experience in collaborative cotherapy with hygiene students and hygiene residents in the experimental program seems to result in a more positive assessment of the role and abilities of dental hygienists, particularly in early detection of abnormalities and in emergency procedures. These results were obtained by the use of an attitude questionnaire distributed to students in all four classes (control and experimental) at the University of Pennsylvania as well as to students from Columbia University and Case Western Reserve dental schools.

Thus it appears that the educational program offered in the Pennsylvania Experiment brings students to a level of achievement at least comparable to that of traditional students at the School of Dental Medicine. At the same time, it offers opportunities for more clinical experiences by students and other educational advantages mentioned above. Also, it has resulted in the acquisition of additional skills and attitudes which should enhance the practice of general dentistry. The evaluation of the educational effects of the experiment should be continued to elaborate further on these findings.

Notes

1. E. H. Porter, *An Introduction to Therapeutic Counseling* (Boston: Houghton Mifflin, 1950).
2. Lewis Bernstein and R. Bernstein, *Interviewing: A Guide for Health Professionals* (New York: Appleton-Century-Crofts, 1980).
3. T. M. Newcomb, "The Prediction of Interpersonal Attraction," *American Psychologists* 11 (1956): 575.
4. Lewis Bernstein and P. E. Veenhuis, "Evaluating a Systematic Approach to Teaching Interviewing," *Journal of Medical Education* 49 (1974): 589.
5. Lewis Bernstein, "Teaching Nurse-Patient Relationships: And Experimental Study," *Nursing Research*, 3 (1954): 80.
6. M. Koslowsky et al., "Satisfaction of the Patient and the Provider: Evaluation by Questionnaire," *Journal of Public Health Dentistry* 34 (1974): 190.
7. C. W. Douglass and J. M. Day, "Cost of Payment of Dental Services in the United States," *Journal of Dental Education* 43 (1979): 330–46.

7

Evaluation, Part II: Financial and Managerial Dimensions, The Busch Center Report

Financial Dimension, Overall Summary

INTRODUCTION

The financial analysis of the Pennsylvania Experiment focused on the following basic questions: Are Models A and B financially viable? Financial viability is defined as the ability to generate sufficient revenue from patient service and tuition monies to cover direct and indirect expenses of operation.

To answer this question, the financial records of Models A and B were analyzed. The results of this analysis are reported in this section.

It must be noted that many changes occurred in the operation of the models over the time period during which the evaluation took place (1980–81, 1981–82). Therefore, these results should be viewed as preliminary; information on the models should be collected over time to ascertain whether the actions of the last two years have significantly affected the financial data.

SUMMARY OF RESULTS

Based on the available data, the following conclusions may be drawn about the financial performance of the models.

Model B

Model B is currently financially viable; it has achieved financial self-sufficiency as a faculty-based private practice and educational unit. Excluding the initial capital investment and startup costs, Model B generated sufficient income to cover its direct expenses, and tuition income was sufficient to cover indirect expenses. Details of the financial operation of Model B are presented in this chapter.

117

It should be noted that Model B's performance is relatively independent of the economics of the rest of the School of Dental Medicine. Because the number of students in Model B is so small (eight clinical and eight preclinical, or only 3 percent of the current total student body at the School of Dental Medicine in 1982), with the current configuration of the School of Dental Medicine and the rules used to allocate its costs, the allocated income and expenses of Model B were not a significant financial factor. Given this current basis of expense allocation, if the proportion of enrollment in Model B increases relative to the student population in the School of Dental Medicine, this independence will decrease.

Based on improvements that occurred in Fiscal Year 1982 (direct income increased about $450,000, while direct expenses increased only $250,000 over Fiscal Year 1981), a surplus of income can be expected in the future, provided the following conditions hold: (1) The productivity levels attained in Fiscal Year 1982 are maintained and improved upon. (In Fiscal Year 1982 productivity increased by 40 percent and total visits to the center increased by 56 percent). (2) Collection of patient collectibles continues. (As of the summer of 1982, there were still $88,000 in patient collectibles and $130,000 in "work-in-progress.") (3) Direct expenses continue to be contained. (For both years of the evaluation, Model B underspent its budget.) (4) The economics of the Penn Faculty Practice Plan continue to be favorable. (This will depend on continued high registration in the plan and on the amount of time the providers devote to its patients. Provider time has increased from approximately 35 percent in the first quarter to about 48 percent in the fourth. If the plan patients' demand for services continues to increase, and no compensating changes are made, it is not likely that surpluses can be sustained.)

Model A

In its present form, Model A is not financially viable. Unlike Model B, in Model A more than half of the income and expenses are allocated from the School of Dental Medicine. Given the magnitude of the costs to the School of Dental Medicine, sufficient revenue cannot be generated to cover these allocated costs. The overall economics of the School of Dental Medicine can significantly alter the performance of Model A.

Managerial improvements made in the third year of the experiment demonstrated that Model A can significantly decrease its deficits through specific actions and further innovations in management, which potentially could lead to financial viability. Some suggested actions follow.

(1) Resident productivity should be increased to $30,000–$35,000, which can be achieved by increasing the number of productive hours and number of visits. Current level of productivity is approximately $19,000. A thorough evaluation of the hygiene program as it relates to the experiment is necessary. The educational benefits of this program must be weighed against its costs. Currently, the hygiene program is not financially viable within the Model A struc-

ture; it will probably require subsidization by the school. (The traditional hygiene program is subsidized in this way.) There should be even further improvements in the productivity of Model A. At the time of this evaluation, the current average was approximately thirty visits per day; this should be increased to forty visits per day. Also, some savings might be realized by using the standard computer system at the School of Dental Medicine.

If Model A is restructured along these lines, it may become a financially viable program to serve as a transition to the Model B environment.

The following pages provide an in-depth analysis of the financial dimensions of Model A and Model B. The financial section also includes a detailed report on the residency program, which generated very promising financial data, and a comparison of student productivity in the models.

Financial Measures

This section provides a detailed description of the activities of the two experimental models during the two evaluation years (July 1, 1980, to June 30, 1982), including details for the second fiscal year (FY82) and comparisons with the first fiscal year (FY81). The available data are categorized and analyzed in the following major categories: financial performance, patient visits, service profile, and provider group performance.

For the purpose of a comparative analysis, the following indicators are selected for each of the above categories.

FINANCIAL PERFORMANCE

- Total income and total expenses for the year

PATIENT VISITS

- Total visits—averages for the year, trends
- Visits breakdown by provider groups
- New patients—averages for the year, trends
- Type of visits
- Cancellations

SERVICE PROFILE

- Percentage of charges generated by each category of services provided
- Chairside hours
- Charges generated by each hour of service in each category

PROVIDER GROUP PERFORMANCE

The following indicators are calculated for each of the provider groups (e.g., faculty, residents, seniors) and averaged for each provider in the group:

- Charges
- Billable charges—equal to charges for dental care minus all adjustments (The reason for adjustments is service fee differentials for the different provider groups, and in Model B for the portion of treatment that is covered by the Penn Faculty Practice Plan.)
- Laboratory costs
- Payments—actual income
- Ratio of income to billable charges
- Total visits
- Billable charges per visit
- Payments per visit
- Total productive time—time spent at chairside with patients
- Visits per productive hour
- Minutes per visit

SOURCES OF DATA

The data used in this analysis are obtained mainly from the Pennsylvania Experiment's computerized Management Information System (MIS) and from the University of Pennsylvania's accounting reports.

Differences between the computer and manual log maintained by the models are noted if they are significant or provide additional information. Other sources of data used are noted in the body of the report. The financial data generated by the models were selectively audited for accuracy and were compared with similar data generated from other sources. Based upon this analysis, the data appear to be representative of the fiscal operation of the models.

FINANCIAL PERFORMANCE

Introduction

There are essentially two types of accounting data available for the analysis of financial performance.

The income and expenses that the university accounting system directly attributed to Models A and B are labeled "direct" income and expense. Direct items are those which are readily indentifiable as having a particular procedure or function. For example, direct costs cover such items as salaries, rent, laboratory costs, and clinic supplies.

The income and expenses which the School of Dental Medicine allocates to each model for that portion of the student's education which takes place outside of the models are labeled "indirect" or "allocated" income and expenses. In this case, indirect items are those which are not readily identifiable with a particular procedure or function. For example, indirect items cover such items as the salaries for basic and clinical sciences faculty and their supporting staff, the general administration of the school, maintenance of buildings, and the tuition income for each model.

Such detailed allocations have been based on the information generated by a financial model developed by Dr. James Galbally and Cecile Feldman.[1] This model uses enrollment and faculty contact hours as its basic allocation parameters.

MODEL B: DENTAL CARE CENTER
Discussion of Model B's Income Statement (Table 7-1)

During the operation in Fiscal Year 1982, Model B generated a surplus of $5,000. Clinic income, which constitutes 91 percent of total Model B income, increased by 75 percent or $400,000 over FY 1981 during the second year (FY82) of analysis. The Pennsylvania Experiment's MIS reports indicate a 100 percent increase from $482,000 to $962,000 as compared to $538,000 and $943,000 for the university reports. This is mainly due to allocation of income to one fiscal year or the other, as the difference in the total income for two years is only $37,000 or about 2 percent between the two sources in FY82.

Direct expenses constitute 95 percent of the total expense. They show an increase of $246,000 (33 percent) in the comparable period. Of this increase, 83 percent was attributable to salaries and benefits, which were 47 percent higher than the year before. Other current expenses rose by only $40,000 (14 percent).

Unless otherwise indicated, the data referred to in this chapter are for FY 1982. All statements about "increases" or "decreases" in financial performance refer to a comparison between these data (FY82) and comparable data from FY 1981.

Currently, the salaries and benefits account for 65 percent of direct expenses.

DETAILS OF OPERATION

VISITS
This section is summarized in Table 7-2.

There were a total of 21,270 visits to the Dental Care Center in Fiscal Year 1982. This total averages to 82.5 patients per day of operation (excluding Saturdays) as compared to 54.8 in FY81 (an increase of 50 percent). This translates into 4.6 visits per chair per day (four additional operatories became available to the center in January 1982, making it a twenty-chair facility) as compared

Table 7-1. Model B: Statement of Income and Expenses, June 30, 1981, to July 1, 1982 (All figures are rounded to nearest thousand)

Income:			
Direct income			
Clinic revenues			
PFP premiums[a]	$366,000		
Patient care	577,000[b]		
		$943,000	
Indirect income			
Tuition[c]	93,000		
Other[d]	3,000		
		96,000	
			$1,039,000
Expenses:			
Direct expenses			
Salaries			
and benefits	$639,000		
Other	343,000		
		$982,000	
Allocated expenses			
Clinical sciences	14,000		
Hospital affairs	8,000		
Program administration	2,000		
Financial aid	4,000		
Net general administration[e]	24,000		
		52,000	
			1,034,000
Surplus (Deficit):			$ 5,000

[a]PFP: Penn Faculty Practice Plan
[b]The patient care total includes copayments for the Penn Faculty Practice Plan.
[c]For eight students at $11,685 each. For the purposes of this analysis, the preclinical students are considered as part of Model A.
[d]Includes special fees and annual giving.
[e]Includes investments, administrative salaries, maintenance of buildings.

to 3.4 visits the year before. The third quarter (January through March) was the busiest quarter with 88 visits per day which is 17 percent higher than the first quarter (July through September), when there were 75 visits per day. Figure 7-1 depicts patient trends during the last two years in Model B.

VISIT BREAKDOWN
As can be observed from the Table 7-3, the general pattern of visits percentage by provider groups was essentially the same during the two years of analysis.

Table 7-2. Model B: Summary of Visits Data

	Total	New	Type of Visit			Cancellations		
			Planned Care	Recall	Acute Care	Canceled Appointments	Broken Appointments	Doctor Rescheduled
FY 1982	21,270	3,434	87%	6%	6%	7%	11%	1%
FY 1981	13,601	1,492	88%	5%	7%	6%	8%	1%
% change	+56	+130	−1	+20	−14	+17	+38	−

	Visits per Day	Visits per Day per Chair	New Patients per Day
FY 1982	+82.5*	4.6*	13.5
FY 1981	55	3.4	6.0
% change	+50	+35	+125

*Excludes the Saturday operation.

Figure 7-1. Model B: Patient Trends

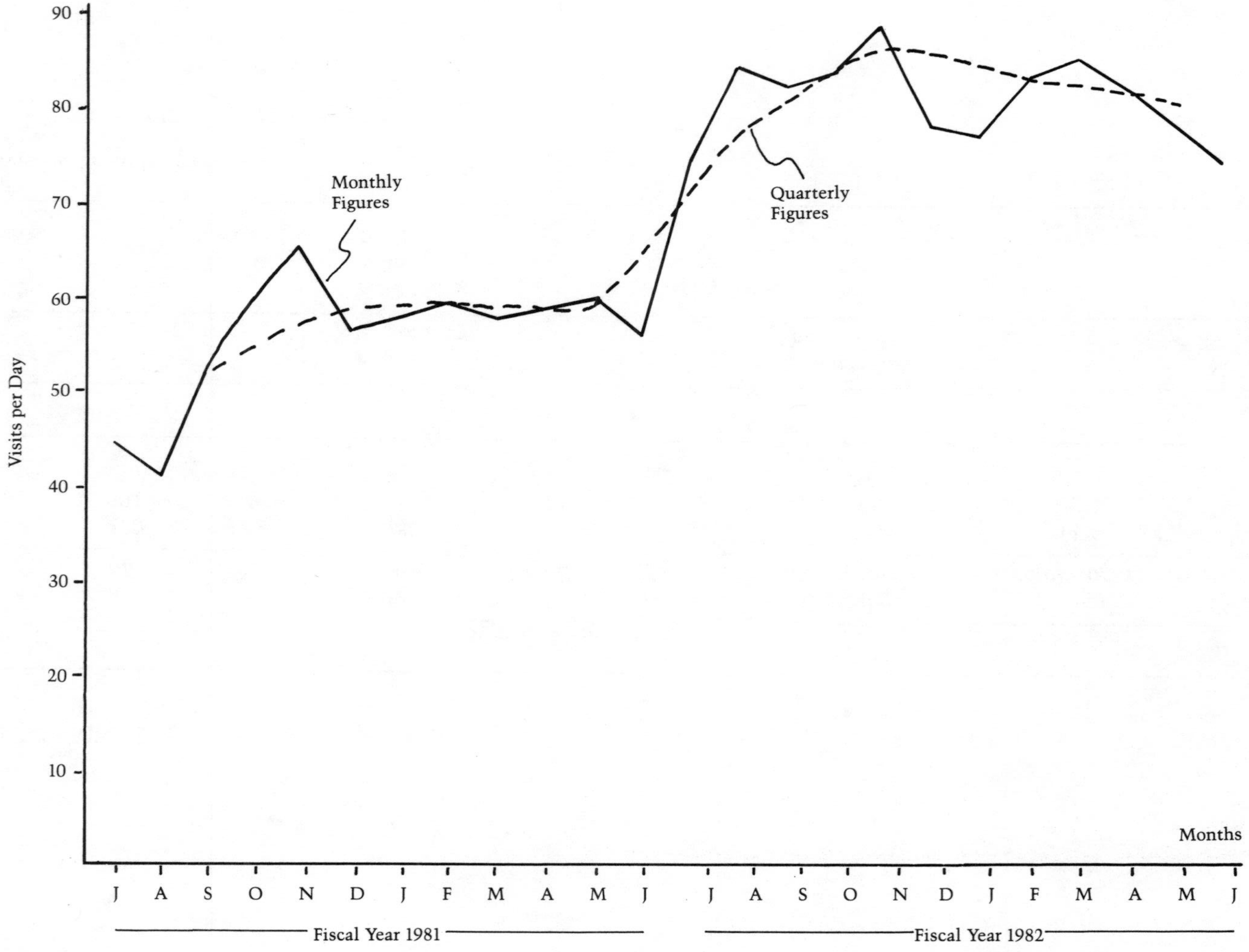

Table 7-3. Model B: Percentage of Visits by Provider Groups

	Full-time Faculty	Part-time Faculty	Hygienists	Residents	Seniors	Juniors	Sophomores
1982:							
Number in group	3.75	8.5	3	4	4	4	4
Total visits	7,283	3,949	4,391	3,665	1,103	837	41
Percent of total	34	19	21	17	5	4	1
1981:							
Number in group	3	8.35	2	3	4	4	4
Total visits	4,081	2,741	2,812	2,010	1,093	837	27
Percent of total	30	20	20	15	8	6	1

NEW PATIENTS

There were a total of 3,434 new patients for the year, or an average of 13.5 per day of operation, which is 125 percent more than the new registrations of the previous year. The trend of new patient registration, however, is downward: from 20 in the first quarter to 8.5 per day in the fourth. The Penn Faculty Practice Plan accounted for 1,591 new patients, or 47 percent of the total. There were 1,849 new patients exclusive of the Penn Faculty Practice Plan, exceeding the total of 1,492 new patients of the previous year (see Figure 7-1).

VISIT TYPES

There has been an increase in percentage of recall visits from the year before. The general pattern, however, is the same as in 1981 (see Table 7-2).

CANCELLATIONS

Broken appointments (canceled without prior notice) and canceled appointments (one-day advance notice) were both higher than the year before. Broken appointments are currently 11 percent, and total cancellations are close to 20 percent of actual visits.

SERVICE PROFILES

Breakdown of service profiles for each provider group are presented in Tables 7-4 and 7-5.

CHAIRSIDE HOURS

The terms "chairside hours" and "productive hours" are used interchangeably throughout this report. The general pattern was the same as in the previous year. There was relatively less time devoted to operative and prosthodontic procedures and more to oral diagnosis, periodontics, and miscellaneous. Table 7-6 summarizes the results.

CHARGES

Charges followed essentially the same pattern of changes as the distribution of hours: percentage charges for operative decreased and those for periodontics, diagnosis, orthodontics, and oral surgery increased.

CHARGES PER HOUR

The general pattern is the same for the two years. The charges per hour are uniformly higher in 1982 even though the fee schedules were the same for the two years. Among the contributing factors are the general increase in the speed of providers (close to 9 percent overall; see Tables 7-7 and 7-8) and the amount of work that has been charged for but is yet to be performed. This second factor, of course, is directly correlated with the increase in the new patients' registration. It is important to note that although there were changes in personnel between the two years, provider mix remained unchanged.

Table 7-4. Model B: Annual Service Profile, 1982, Productive Hours

Group	Oral Diagnosis	Prevention	Periodontics	Restorative (no lab)	Restorative (lab)	Fixed Prosthetics	Removable Prosthetics	Endodontics	Orthodontics	Oral Surgery	Miscellaneous
Full-time faculty	418 8.0%*	50 0.1%	365 6.6%	2,168 39.4%	833 15.2%	433 7.9%	184 3.3%	308 5.6%	76 1.4%	187 3.4%	475 8.6%
Part-time faculty	330 9.8%	69 2.0%	153 4.5%	710 21.0%	313 9.3%	31 0.9%	190 5.6%	472 14.0%	299 8.9%	215 6.4%	594 17.6%
Hygienists**	1,143 27.9%	1,529 37.3%	1,371 33.4%	2 0%	– –	– –	– –	– –	– –	– –	56 1.4%
Residents	537 15.4%	85 2.4%	322 9.2%	988 28.3%	443 12.7%	97 2.8%	170 4.9%	483 13.8%	13 0.4%	106 3.0%	252 7.2%
Seniors	111 6.4%	77 4.4%	160 9.2%	387 22.3%	331 19.0%	101 5.8%	255 14.7%	188 10.8%	24 1.4%	28 1.6%	76 4.4%
Juniors	156 12.3%	108 8.5%	140 11.0%	443 34.8%	111 8.7%	48 3.8%	86 6.8%	130 10.2%	– –	22 1.7%	28 2.2%
Sophomores	24 27.3%	15 17.0%	30 34.1%	17 19.3%	– –	– –	– –	– –	– –	2 2.3%	– –
Model B TOTAL	2,719 13.9%	1,933 9.9%	2,541 12.9%	4,715 24.1%	2,031 10.4%	710 3.6%	885 4.5%	1,581 8.1%	412 2.1%	560 2.9%	1,481 7.6%

*In each cell the top number is the total number of hours devoted to a service category and the second number is the percentage of time devoted to that category by the provider group (i.e., row total = 100%). Dashes indicate no activity in a service category by the provider group.

**Includes hygiene resident.

Table 7-5. Model B: Annual Service Profile, 1982, Charges

Group	Oral Diagnosis	Prevention	Periodontics	Restorative (no lab)	Restorative (lab)	Fixed Prosthetics	Removable Prosthetics	Endodontics	Orthodontics	Oral Surgery	Miscellaneous
Full-time faculty	$16,444 3%*	$ 2,225 0%	$ 49,650 10%	$130,310 27%	$121,385 25%	$ 87,479 18%	$ 31,164 6%	$ 29,440 6%	$ 4,715 1%	$11,740 2%	$ 2,790 1%
Part-time faculty	10,755 4%	2,950 1%	19,370 7%	36,440 13%	62,025 22%	10,475 4%	28,559 10%	49,060 17%	41,240 14%	18,800 7%	4,800 2%
Hygienists**	46,412 27%	56,621 33%	66,835 39%	110 0%	– –	– –	– –	– –	– –	– –	400 1%
Residents	16,138 8%	5,501 3%	20,675 10%	45,520 22%	38,410 19%	12,760 6%	20,620 10%	32,900 16%	235 0%	5,945 3%	3,896 2%
Seniors	2,180 3%	1,407 2%	9,655 12%	10,300 13%	19,120 25%	9,200 12%	17,120 22%	6,675 9%	505 1%	1,280 2%	125 0%
Juniors	2,323 4%	2,392 4%	7,165 13%	9,700 18%	10,130 19%	8,125 15%	7,310 13%	6,105 11%	– –	1,300 2%	85 0%
Sophomores	226 14%	210 13%	775 49%	210 13%	– –	– –	– –	– –	– –	160 10%	– –
Model B TOTAL	$94,478 7.4%	$71,306 5.6%	$174,125 13.6%	$232,590 18.2%	$251,070 19.6%	$128,039 10.0%	$104,773 8.2%	$124,180 9.7%	$46,695 3.7%	$39,225 3.1%	$12,096 0.9%

*In each cell the top number is the total charges for a service category and the second number is the percentage of charges for that category by the provider group (i.e., row total). Dashes indicate no activity in a service category by the provider group.

**Includes hygiene resident.

Table 7-6. Model B: Chairside Hours (percentages)

	1982	1981
Operative*	34.5	39.5
Oral diagnosis	13.9	12.0
Periodontics	12.9	12.2
Preventive	9.9	10.2
Endodontics	8.1	8.2
Removable prosthetics	4.5	5.1
Fixed prosthetics	3.6	4.9
Oral surgery	2.9	1.9
Orthodontics	2.1	2.1
Miscellaneous	7.6	4.4

*Operative procedures includes restorative procedures with or without lab.

Table 7-7. Model B: Charges (percentages)

	1982	1981
Operative*	37.8	40.5
Periodontics	13.6	12.6
Fixed prosthetics	10.0	9.7
Endodontics	9.7	9.7
Removable prosthetics	8.2	8.1
Oral diagnosis	8.2	8.1
Preventive	5.6	5.2
Orthodontics	3.7	2.6
Oral surgery	3.1	1.7
Miscellaneous	.9	.7

*Operative procedures include restorative procedures with or without lab.

PROVIDER GROUP PERFORMANCE

This section is summarized in Table 7-9. Some highlights and additional information are presented below. All the figures in this section should be regarded as approximations because of the allocation decisions made for the capitation premiums and MIS inconsistencies.

FULL-TIME FACULTY

The average faculty member generated $100,000 in income, completed close to 2,000 visits, and spent 1,400 hours at chairside delivering care while also

Table 7-8. Model B: Charges per Hour

	1982	1981
Fixed prosthetics	$180.34	$143.35
Restorative with lab	123.62	94.97
Removable prosthetics	118.39	88.15
Orthodontics	113.34	67.92
Endodontics	78.55	66.65
Oral surgery	70.04	50.10
Periodontics	68.53	57.98
Restorative without lab	49.33	40.73
Preventive	36.89	31.53
Oral diagnosis	34.75	30.34
Miscellaneous	8.17	7.19

instructing residents and students. This is an impressive overall improvement in performance as compared to 1981: visits per person increased by 43 percent, productive hours increased by 33 percent, and payments were 51 percent higher. Laboratory charges per visit were 8 percent lower, and billable charges per visit decreased by 13 percent.

PART-TIME FACULTY

The same general pattern of overall improvement in performance is evident: 42 percent increase in visits, 36 percent increase in productive hours, and 66 percent increase in payments and charges. During the course of the year more than ten part-time members were involved with the model. Their hours were equivalent to 2.75 full-time faculty. The income generated by the group was $25,000 per person or $76,000 per full-time equivalent. Visits were slightly more than 1,400 per FTE.

HYGIENE

Average payments for each hygienist's services doubled in 1982. Billable charges per visit also increased by 46 percent. There were two experienced hygiene faculty and a first-year hygiene resident in this group. The hygiene resident did not work in the clinic for more than four days per week. Thus her performance was lower than that of the hygiene faculty, as Table 7-10 indicates. If the figures are adjusted for the additional work day, however, the hygiene resident has had an impressive performance at the same level of more experienced hygienists.

If only the performance of hygiene faculty is compared to their 1981 performance, there are even higher improvements: payments increased by 123 percent, productive hours increased by 8 percent, and visits increased by 9 percent.

Table 7-9. Model B: Annual Activity Summary by Provider Groups, 1982*

Provider Group	Charges ($)	Billable Charges ($)	Lab Charges ($)	Pay-ments ($)	Payments to Billable (%)	Visits	Billable Charges per Visit	Lab Charges per Visit	Payments per Visit	Productive Hours	Minutes per Visit
Full-time faculty (N = 3.75)	479,197	374,941	53,443	374,471	100%	7,283	51.48	7.34	51.42	5,365	44
	127,786	99,984	14,251	99,859		1,942				1,431	
	+29%	+24%	+31%	+51%	+22%	+43%	−13%	−8%	+6%	+33%	−8%
Part-time faculty (N = 8.5)	280,940	243,567	18,136	209,751	86%	3,949	61.68	4.59	53.11	3,318	50
	33,052	28,655	2,134	24,677		465				390	
	+65%	+54%	+11%	+66%	+8%	+42%	+9%	−22%	+18%	+36%	−6%
Hygienists (N = 3)	164,418	157,270	NA	159,595	101%	4,391	35.81	NA	36.35	3,962	54
	54,806	52,423		53,198		1,464				1,321	
	+18%	+52%		+101%	+33%	+4%	+46%		+93%	0	−5%
Residents (N = 4)	199,930	154,238	14,341	147,106	95%	3,665	42.08	3.91	40.14	3,567	58
	49,983	38,560	3,585	36,777		916					
	+63%	+75%	+18%	+89%	+8%	+37%	+28%	−13%	+38%	+33%	−3%
Seniors (N = 4)	77,567	48,195	6,400	47,245	98%	1,103	43.69	5.80	42.83	1,735	94
	19,392	12,049	1,600	11,811		276				434	
	0	+29%	−29%	+50%	+17%	0	+27%	−30%	+49%	−8%	−10%
Juniors (N = 4)	54,635	32,234	1,893	23,328	72%	837	38.51	2.26	27.87	1,281	91
	13,659	8,059	473	5,832		209				320	
	−10%	+58%	+2%	+44%	−10%	0	+58%	+2%	+44%	−16%	−17%
Sophomores (N = 4)	1,631	500	NA	396	79%	41	12.20	NA	9.66	97	142
	414	125		99		27				68	
	−29%	−57%		−37%	+46%	+43%	−72%		−58%	+41%	−3%
TOTAL Dental Care Center	1,258,318	1,010,945	94,213	961,868	95%	21,270	47.53	4.43	45.22	19,324	55
	+62%	+71%	+37%	+100%	+17%	+56%	+9%	−12%	+28%	+40%	−9%

* Top line in table shows total for each group, second line is the average for each provider in the group, and third line is percentage change per provider from previous year.

Table 7-10. Model B: Hygiene Service Profile

	Charges	Billable Charges	Payments	Visits	Productive Hours
Hygiene resident	$48,000	$49,000	$44,000	1,300	1,200
Average for other hygienists	60,000	56,000	58,000	1,600	1,400

RESIDENTS

The improvement in resident productivity has been very impressive. Each resident generated close to $38,000 in revenues. Charges per resident increased by 63 percent, visits by 37 percent, productive hours by 33 percent, and payments by 89 percent. The PFP allocation accounts for about $16,500 for each resident. Without any PFP allocation, the residents generated more income per person than the year before ($20,300 versus $19,500).

SENIORS

Productive hours declined by 8 percent, but the number of visits and total charges remained the same. The major differences were in payments, which increased by 50 percent, and laboratory charges, which declined by 30 percent.

Each senior student generated close to $12,000 in clinic income.

JUNIORS

For the juniors, productive hours declined by 16 percent, and visits remained at the same level. The major differences were in billable charges (increase of 58 percent) and payments (increase of 44 percent).

Each junior student generated close to $6,000 in clinic income.

SOPHOMORES

The number of visits increased from 27 in 1981 to 41 in 1982 for the group as a whole, and productive hours went from 68 to 97. The charges and payments, however, were lower than Fiscal Year 1982.

MODEL B TOTAL

The Dental Care Center had a very impressive year in Fiscal Year 1982. Productive hours increased by 40 percent and visits by 56 percent from FY81. The payments doubled in 1982; their ratio to billable charges increased by 17 percent and total charges increased by 62 percent. The Dental Care Center delivered 20,000 hours of dental care to the community and produced close to $950,000 in clinical revenues. Direct expenses were about $980,000. Tuition income was over $90,000.

Model A: Paletz Clinic

DISCUSSION OF MODEL A'S INCOME STATEMENT (TABLE 7–11)

The operation of Model A in Fiscal Year 1982 resulted in a deficit of $194,000. Clinic income, however, which constitutes 33 percent of total Model A income, increased by 37 percent over the previous fiscal year (FY81). According to the Pennsylvania Experiment computer reports, the Model A income increase was approximately 50 percent. The university reports income of

Table 7-11. Model A: Statement of Income and Expenses, June 30, 1981 to July 1, 1982 (All figures are rounded to nearest thousand)

Income:				
Direct income				
Clinic revenues			$266,000	
Indirect income				
Tuition[a]				
D.M.D.	$456,000			
Hygiene	46,000			
		$502,000		
Other				
Radiology and admissions	16,000			
Special fee and annual giving	18,000			
		34,000		
			536,000	
				$ 802,000
Expenses:				
Direct expenses				
Salaries and benefits	$393,000			
Other	136,000			
			$529,000	
Allocated expenses				
Basic sciences	82,000			
Clinical sciences	139,000			
Radiology and admissions	60,000			
Hospital affairs	15,000			
Program administration	8,000			
Financial aid	20,000			
Net general administration[b]	143,000			
			467,000	
				$ 996,000
Surplus (deficit):				$(194,000)

[a]For thirty-nine D.M.D. students at $11,685 each, including the eight students who will continue their clinical education at Model B and eight Hygiene students at $5,790 each.

[b]Includes investments, administrative salaries, and maintenance of buildings.

$194,000 and $266,000 for the two years, as compared to $170,000 and $262,000 for the MIS reports.

In the comparable period, direct expenses, which constitute 53 percent of total expenses, increased by 24 percent from $427,000 to $529,000. The increase in direct expenses is solely owing to salaries and employee benefits, which increased by $115,000 (41 percent) while other expenses declined by $12,000 (8 percent), mainly because of reduced laboratory costs.

Salaries and benefits constitute 75 percent of direct expenses.

DETAILS OF OPERATION

VISITS
This section is summarized in Table 7-12.

TOTAL VISITS
Visits to the Paletz Clinic totaled 7,373 (the manual log shows a total of 7,395, or .2 percent difference) for Fiscal Year 1982, which averages to about 30 visits per day of operation (there were 248 days of operation in FY82), or 2 visits per chair per day (there are fifteen chairs in the clinic). These figures show a one-third increase over the comparable period, FY81. The second quarter (October through December 1981) was the busiest quarter of the year, with close to 33 visits per day, while the fourth quarter was the lowest in this regard, with 27 visits per day. Figure 7-2 depicts the patient trends for Model A for the past two years.

VISIT BREAKDOWN
The hygiene resident, who was added to Model A in September 1981, accounted for 7 percent of total visits, and the D.M.D. residents accounted for 46 percent. Table 7-13 summarizes the percentage of visits by each provider group.

NEW PATIENTS
The new patient registration totaled 1,324, as compared with 1,257 for the year before. For each day of operation, there were approximately 5.3 new patients (see Table 7-12 and Figure 7-2).

VISIT TYPES
Recall visits increased to 520, compared to 330 the year before, to account for 7 percent of visits to the clinic. The breakdown of visit types is very similar to the year before except for the increase in recalls. Emergency visits are 12 percent and 81 percent are planned care (see Table 7-12).

CANCELLATIONS
Broken appointments (canceled without prior notice) continued to be high at 9 percent of total visits. In the second year, there was a decline in canceled

Table 7-12. Model A: Summary of Visits Data

		Type of Visit				Cancellations	
	New Patients	Planned Care	Recall	Acute Care	Canceled Appointments	Broken Appointments	Doctor Rescheduled
Total Visits							
FY 1982	7,373	1,324	81%	7%	12%	1%	9%	1%
FY 1981	5,514	1,257	83%	6%	12%	3%	9%	2%
% change	+34	+5	-2	+2		67	-50	

	Visits per Day	Visits per Day per Chair	New Patients per Day
FY 1982	30	2.0	5.3
FY 1981	23	1.5	5.2
% change	+31	+31	+3

Figure 7-2. Model A: Patient Trends

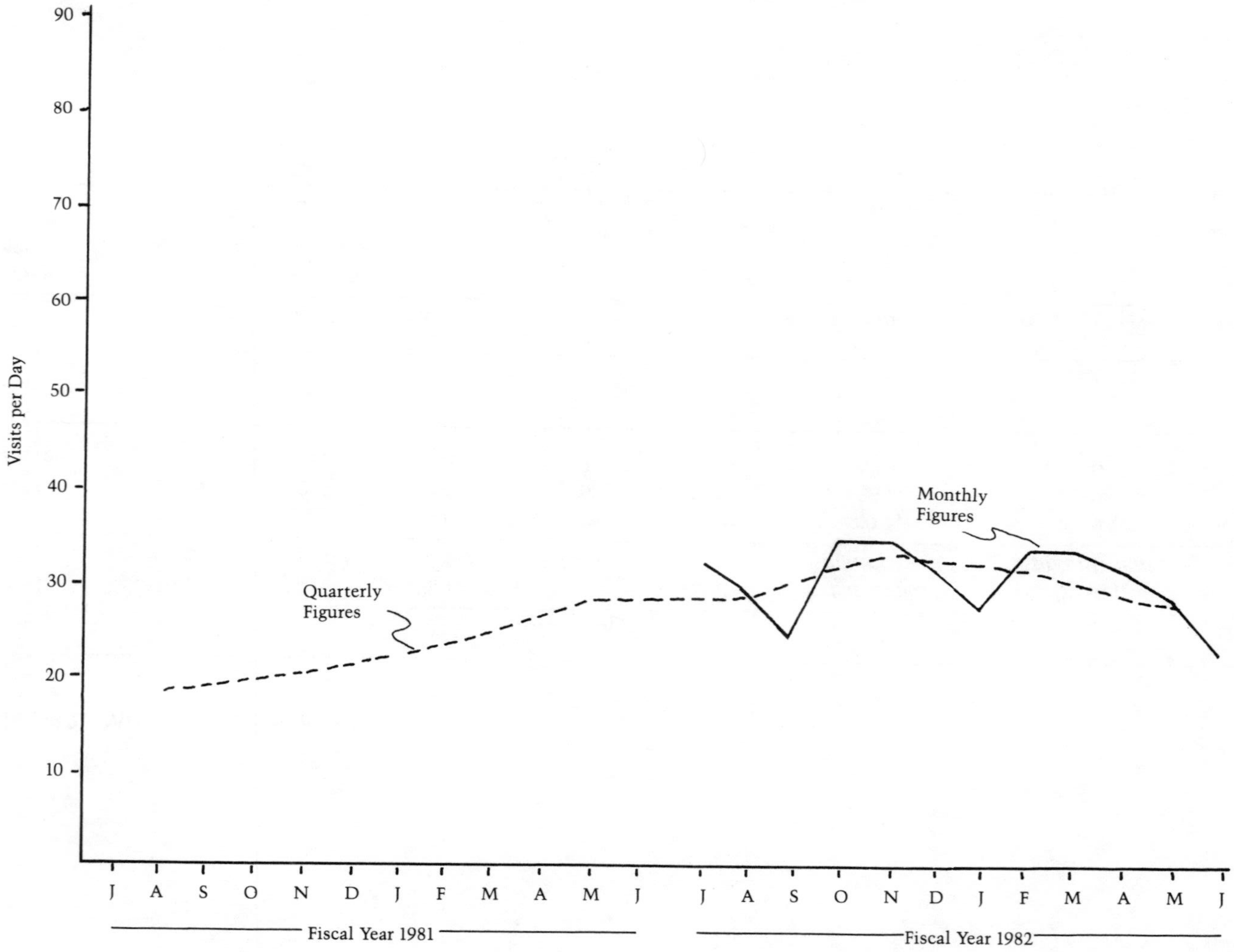

Table 7-13. Model A: Percentage of Visits by Provider Groups

	Residents	Seniors	Juniors	Sophomores	Hygiene Resident	Second-year Hygiene	First-year Hygiene
1982:							
Number in group	8	7	8	8	1	4	4
Total visits	3,410	1,378	1,592	97	498	327	70
Percent of total	46	19	22	1	7	4	1
1981:							
Number in group	5.5	6	6	7	—	4.25	4
Total visits	1,854	1,598	1,333	165	—	478	86
Percent of total	34	29	24	3	—	9	1

appointments (at least twenty-four-hour notice) and doctor-rescheduled appointments each at 1 percent of total visits (see Table 7-12).

SERVICE PROFILE
This section is summarized in Tables 7-14 and 7-15.

CHAIRSIDE HOURS
There was a shift of pattern in service breakdown in 1982 compared to 1981. More time was spent in prevention, operative, and, to a small extent, periodontics and less time in fixed prosthetics and oral diagnosis. Table 7-14 provides a comparison of the patterns for the two years. Actual number of hours and breakdown by provider groups are reported in Tables 7-14 and 7-16.

CHARGES
The pattern of shift in charges is parallel to that of chairside hours: less fixed prosthetics, more periodontics, and more operative (see Table 7-17).

PROVIDER GROUP PERFORMANCE
This section is summarized in Table 7-18. Some highlights and additional information are presented below. All figures in this section and in Table 7-18 are approximations because of inconsistencies in the MIS report.

RESIDENTS
Each resident spent almost one-third more time chairside in 1982 and had one-third more visits than the year before. Although billable charges were the same ($22,000 per person), payments increased by 20 percent ($18,000), and laboratory charges were reduced by 50 percent. The decrease of billable charges per visit and laboratory charges per visit can be attributed to a shift in pattern of services: fixed prosthetics accounted for 19 percent of chairside hours of residents in 1981 but for less than 10 percent of hours in 1982. Percentage of hours in operative procedures, periodontics, and removable prosthetics increased over the year before.

The residency program includes three months of hospital rotation time and two weeks of vacation. Hence all the figures are for only eight and one-half months of clinical work per resident.

SENIORS
There was a 27 percent decline in productive hours and visits per senior in Fiscal Year 1982 as compared to the year before. This reduction is in part because the seniors had less chairtime available in 1982 because the total number of students increased over 1981. Payments per visit, however, increased by 20 percent, principally because of a much improved ratio of payments to billable charges (94 percent in 1982 as compared to 60 percent in 1981).

Charges of $12,000 per senior were 43 percent smaller than 1981. The sec-

Table 7-14. Model A: Annual Service Profile, Productive Hours*

Group	Oral Diagnosis	Prevention	Periodontics	Restorative (no lab)	Restorative (lab)	Fixed Prosthetics	Removable Prosthetics	Endodontics	Orthodontics	Oral Surgery	Miscellaneous
Residents	485	54	392	975	1,177	503	339	310	86	59	717
	9.5%	1.1%	7.7%	19.1%	23.1%	9.9%	6.7%	6.1%	1.7%	1.2%	14.1%
Seniors	139	66	163	609	371	308	397	108	15	52	69
	5.9%	2.8%	6.9%	25.8%	15.7%	13.1%	16.8%	7.2%	0.6%	2.9%	3.4%
Juniors	471	321	360	1,168	363	112	178	277	22	60	75
	13.8%	9.4%	10.6%	34.3%	10.7%	3.3%	5.2%	8.1%	0.6%	1.8%	2.2%
Sophomores	89	35	39	44	8	–	3	3	–	5	2
	39.3%	15.7%	17.1%	19.7%	3.4%	–	1.1%	1.1%	–	2.1%	0.7%
Hygiene resident	18	324	156	4	–	–	–	–	–	–	1
	3.5%	64.5%	31.0%	0.8%	–	–	–	–	–	–	0.2%
Second-year hygienists	205	501	55	–	–	–	–	–	–	–	–
	26.9%	65.9%	7.2%	–	–	–	–	–	–	–	–
First-year hygienists	2	190	–	–	–	–	–	–	–	–	–
	0.8%	99.2%	–	–	–	–	–	–	–	–	–
Model A TOTAL	1,409	1,490	1,164	2,800	1,919	922	916	760	123	176	864
	11.2%	11.9%	9.3%	22.3%	15.3%	7.4%	7.3%	6.1%	1.0%	1.4%	6.9%

* The number in the top line in the table is the total number of hours devoted to a service category and the number in the second line is the percentage of time devoted to that category by the provider group (i.e., line total = 100%). Dashes indicate no activity in a service category by the provider group.

Table 7-15. Model A: Annual Service Profile, Charges*

Group	Oral Diagnosis	Prevention	Periodontics	Restorative (no lab)	Restorative (lab)	Fixed Prosthetics	Removable Prosthetics	Endodontics	Orthodontics	Oral Surgery	Miscellaneous
Residents	$ 4,331 2.1%	$ 1,313 0.6%	$ 16,920 8.0%	$26,762 12.6%	$ 68,510 32.4%	$50,455 23.8%	$17,647 8.3%	$11,645 5.5%	$2,580 1.2%	$2,126 1.0%	$ 9,468 4.5%
Seniors	1,549 1.8%	1,114 1.3%	83,825 9.7%	13,278 15.8%	17,460 20.8%	19,775 23.5%	13,745 16.3%	5,740 6.8%	405 0.5%	1,944 2.3%	723 0.7%
Juniors	3,747 4.8%	3,370 4.3%	10,870 13.8%	15,490 19.6%	18,330 23.2%	7,955 10.1%	9,340 11.8%	6,710 8.5%	675 0.9%	2,142 2.7%	325 0.4%
Sophomores	709 20.3%	300 8.6%	1,235 35.4%	475 13.6%	605 17.3%	–	50 1.4%	15 0.4%	–	86 2.5%	15 0.4%
Hygiene resident	349 2.2%	7,835 50.0%	7,420 47.4%	50 0.3%	–	–	–	–	–	–	15 0.01%
Second-year hygienists	1,422 20.8%	4,933 72.1%	490 7.2%	–	–	–	–	–	–	–	–
First-year hygienists	–	7,190 100%	–	–	–	–	–	–	–	–	–
Model A TOTAL	$12,107 3.0%	$19,584 4.9%	$453,175 11.3%	$56,055 14.0%	$104,905 26.1%	$78,185 19.5%	$40,782 10.2%	$24,110 6.0%	$3,660 0.9%	$6,289 1.6%	$10,546 2.6%

*The number in the top line in the table is the total number of hours devoted for a service category and the number in the second line is the percentage of charges for that category by the provider group (i.e., line total = 100%). Dashes indicate no activity in a service category by the provider group.

Table 7-16. Model A: Chairside Hours (percentages)

	1982	1981
Operative*	37.6	35.7
Preventive	11.9	8.5
Oral diagnosis	11.2	16.1
Periodontics	9.3	8.5
Fixed prosthetics	7.4	9.8
Removable prosthetics	7.3	7.3
Endodontics	6.1	6.2
Oral surgery	1.4	1.0
Orthodontics	1.0	.8
Miscellaneous	6.9	4.8

Table 7-17. Model A: Total Charges (percentages)

	1982	1981
Operative*	40.2	37.8
Fixed prosthetics	19.5	25.6
Periodontics	11.3	9.1
Removable prosthetics	10.2	10.8
Endodontics	6.0	5.6
Preventive	4.9	3.4
Oral diagnosis	3.0	4.1
Oral surgery	1.6	0.8
Orthodontics	0.9	0.5
Miscellaneous	2.6	2.0

*Operative procedures include restorative procedures with or without lab.

ond quarter was the period with highest charges, at the annual rate of $21,000 per person, but the rate for first and fourth quarters was only $6,500 per person.

JUNIORS
Payments and payments per visit increased dramatically (over 50 percent) for the average junior. The ratio of payments to billable charges increased from 61 to 96 percent. They also spent 15 percent more time chairside than the year before but had fewer visits. This is perhaps because of a change of pattern in the service profile. Each junior spent fourteen hours in fixed prosthetics in

Table 7-18. Model A: Annual Activity Summary by Provider Groups, 1982*

Provider Group	Charges ($)	Billable Charges ($)	Lab Charges ($)	Payments ($)	Payments to Billable (%)	Visits	Billable Charges per Visit	Lab Charges per Visit	Payments per Visit	Productive Hours	Minutes per Visit
Residents (N = 8)	211,757	176,491	31,872	144,146	82%	3,410	51.76	9.35	42.27	5,098	90
	26,470	22,061	3,984	18,018		426				637	
	+12%	0	−49%	+19%	+19%	+30%	−21%	−60%	−6%	+29%	+2%
Seniors (N = 7)	84,115	60,709	10,669	57,354	94%	1,378	44.09	7.75	41.75	2,358	103
	12,016	8,673	1,524	8,193		197				337	
	−43%	−43%	−63%	−11%	+57%	+26%	−23%	−50%	+21%	+27%	+1%
Juniors (N = 8)	78,954	51,893	3,299	49,623	96%	1,592	32.60	2.07	31.17	3,405	128
	9,869	6,487	412	6,203		199				426	
	+5%	−2%	+159%	+53%	+57%	−7%	+5%	+176%	+64%	+15%	+22%
Sophomores (N = 8)	3,490	1,940	NA	955	49%	97	20.00	NA	9.85	225	139
	436	243		119		12				28	
	−47%	−40%		−67%	−46%	−50%	+17%		−37%	−44%	+11%
Hygiene resident (N = 1)	15,867	11,297	NA	7,230	64%	498	22.68	NA	14.52	519	63
Second-year hygiene (N = 4)	6,647	3,809	NA	2,161	57%	327	11.65	NA	6.61	743	136
	1,662	952		540		18				186	
	−18%	−39%		−46%	−11%	−27%	−16%		−26%	−22%	+6%
First-year hygiene (N = 4)	719	557	NA	236	42%	70	7.96	NA	3.37	191	164
	186	139		56		82				186	
	−50%	−27%		−54%	−38%	−18%	−10%		−43%	−21%	−4%
TOTAL Paletz Clinic	401,549	306,699	45,840	261,706	85%	7,373	41.60	6.22	35.50	12,539	102
	+21%	+16%	−34%	+53%	+31%	+34%	−13%	−50%	+15%	+33%	0

*Top line shows total for each group, second line is the average for each provider in the group, and third line is percentage change per provider from previous year.

1982 as compared to eight hours in 1981. Thus the laboratory charges increased significantly. This is the first class to have completed its preclinical education in the experimental setting, suggesting that they can start more complicated procedures earlier in their clinical years.

Billable charges were at the same level as the year before, at $6,500 per person. The pattern of quarterly charges was the same as last year. Third and fourth quarter charges were at an annual rate of about $14,000.

SOPHOMORES
There was an overall decline in the productivity data for sophomores with the exception of billable charges per visit, which increased from $17 to $20. This is partly because less chair time was available to them because of an increase in the number of upperclasspersons and residents in the clinic.

HYGIENE RESIDENT
This was an additional provider group in Model A which did not exist in 1981. There was one hygiene resident who worked for 520 productive hours, producing $11,300 in billable charges. The actual payments were low, at $7,200. On the average, each visit took 63 minutes.

HYGIENE
There was an overall decline for both hygiene classes. A poor collection rate led to a total of $2,300 income for both classes combined. The two classes spent 950 hours chairside, completing about 400 visits. In 1981 the comparable group collected $4,700 for 1,200 productive hours.

MODEL A TOTAL
Overall, this was a growth year for the Paletz Clinic (Model A). Productive hours and number of visits increased by 33 percent over 1981, while the payments increased by 53 percent. Laboratory charges were 34 percent lower and the payments to billable ratio increased by 31 percent.

Direct expenses for the same period increased by 24 percent to $530,000 while total clinic income increased to about $270,000.

The Residency Program

INTRODUCTION
The fifth-year General Practice Residency Program, which began in July 1979, is an integral part of the Pennsylvania Experiment. The program includes four days of clinical work per week and one day for teaching and preparation of reports and papers. It also includes three months of hospital rotation and two weeks of vacation.

The following sections provide the details of clinical productivity of the residents in the two models during the two evaluation years.

Table 7-19. Model B: Residents

	1982	1981	% Change
Charges	$49,983.00	$30,657.00	+63
Billable charges	38,560.00	22,057.00	+75
Payments	36,777.00	19,500.00	+89
Lab charges	3,585.00	3,030.00	+18
Visits	916.00	670.00	+37
Productive hours	892.00	669.00	+33
Billable charges per visit	42.08	32.92	+28
Lab charges per visit	3.91	4.52	−13
Payments per visit	40.14	29.11	+38

MODEL B

There has been an impressive improvement in the performance of Model B residents during the two years of evaluation, as Table 7-19 demonstrates.

The increase in average income, from $19,500 to $36,800, is especially noteworthy. This level of production has been achieved in eight and a half months, with four days of clinical work, which is equivalent to over $60,000 for a full-time resident (forty hours per week and no hospital rotation).

The average resident spent 41 percent of his or her time on Penn Faculty Practice Plan patients. The allocation of PFP premiums was $16,500 for each resident.

SERVICE PROFILE

There was a shift from concentration on operative and prosthetic procedures in FY81 to more periodontics and prevention in FY82. During 1981, the residents spent 64 percent of their time in operative and prosthodontics, compared to 48 percent in 1982, and 17 percent on periodontics, prevention, and oral diagnosis in 1981 as compared to 27 percent in 1982.

The residents spent more time in almost every category of service in 1982 compared to 1981, as Table 7-20 indicates.

MODEL A

The income generated by each resident in Model A increased by about $3,000 between the first and second years of evaluation. The most significant change, however, has been the reduction of laboratory charges by 50 percent and of laboratory charges per visit by 60 percent. This decline is mostly a result of a shift in the pattern of services with relatively less emphasis on prosthodontics during 1982. Table 7-21 summarizes other changes.

The decrease in billable charges per visit occurred partly because some of the work that was charged in 1981 was actually performed in 1982 and partly because of the shift in the service profile toward less costly procedures.

Table 7-20. Residents in Model B: Average Chairside Hours per Person

	1982	1981
Oral diagnosis and prevention	156	80
Periodontics	81	32
Operative*	358	320
Prosthodontics	67	100
Endodontics	121	72
Orthodontics	3	6
Oral surgery	27	22
Other	63	26

*Includes restorative procedures with or without lab.

Table 7-21. Model A: Residents

	1982	1981	% Change
Charges	$26,470.00	$23,638.00	+12
Billable charges	22,061.00	22,007.00	0
Payments	18,018.00	15,087.00	+19
Lab charges	3,984.00	7,888.00	−49
Visits	426.00	337.00	+30
Productive hours	637.00	493.00	+29
Billable charges per visit	51.76	65.30	−21
Lab charges per visit	9.35	23.40	−60
Payments per visit	42.27	44.76	−6

SERVICE PROFILE

Table 7-22 summarizes the service profile for the two years.

The proportion of hours spent on prosthodontics decreased from 24 percent in 1981 to 16 percent in 1982, while the operative procedures increased from 37 percent to 42 percent during the same period. Periodontal procedures in 1982 constituted 8 percent of total chairside hours, as compared to 5 percent in 1981. In absolute numbers, this change is much more significant: from 21 hours per resident in 1981 to 49 hours in 1982. Operative procedures also increased significantly, from 180 to 270 hours in 1982.

COMPARISON AND CONCLUSIONS

Analysis of the two years of evaluation leads to the following conclusions about Models A and B. Model B residents generate more income than Model A residents (see Table 7-23). This difference has substantially increased during 1982 and is most pronounced in payments. Table 7-24 provides more details.

Table 7-22. Residents in Model A: Average
Chairside Hours per Person

	1982	1981
Oral diagnosis and pre-vention	67	62
Periodontics	49	21
Operative*	269	183
Prosthodontics	105	118
Endodontics	39	31
Orthodontics	11	8
Oral surgery	7	6
Other	90	60

*Includes restorative procedures with or without lab.

Table 7-23. Model A and Model B: Comparison of
Resident Income

	Average Payments	Billable Charges
1982:		
Model B	36,777	38,559
Model A	18,018	22,061
% difference*	204	175
1981:		
Model B	19,500	22,057
Model A	15,087	22,007
% difference*	129	0

*These differences represent Model B's figures as a percentage
of Model A's.

Although payments per visit and billable charges per visit are higher for
Model A residents, so are the lab charges per visit. Thus payments minus lab
charges per visit are still higher for Model B residents (see Table 7-25).

The reason for the difference in lab charges is the difference in the service
profile.

Model B residents spend more time chairside and complete more visits than
Model A residents.

As Table 7-26 shows, this difference is remarkable and increased slightly in
1982.

Table 7-24. Model A and Model B: Comparison of Resident Income

	Billable Charges per Visit	Payments per Visit	Lab Charges per Visit
1982:			
Model B	42.08	40.14	3.91
Model A	51.76	42.27	9.35
% difference*	81	95	42
1981:			
Model B	32.92	29.11	4.52
Model A	65.30	44.76	23.40
% difference*	50	65	19

* These differences represent Model B's figures as a percentage of Model A's.

Table 7-25. Model A and Model B: Payments Minus Lab Charges per Visit (Residents)

	1982	1981
Model B	$36.23	$24.59
Model A	32.92	21.36

Table 7-26. Model A and Model B: Number of Visits and Productive Hours (Residents)

	Visits	Productive Hours
1982:		
Model B	916	892
Model A	426	637
% difference*	215	140
1981:		
Model B	670	669
Model A	337	493
% difference*	199	136

* These differences represent Model B's figures as a percentage of Model A's.

An average visit takes about one hour for Model B residents and one and a half hours for Model A residents.

Also, the relative emphasis on the various service categories is different for the two models.

Model A residents spend relatively more time on fixed and removable prosthetics, restorative procedures with lab (inlays, onlays, and the like), orthodontics, and miscellaneous procedures. Model B residents devote more time to diagnosis, prevention, periodontics, simple restorative procedures, endodontics, and oral surgery (see Table 7-27).

In absolute number of hours, however, Model B residents spend more time on every category of care except for prosthodontics, orthodontics, and miscellaneous procedures. Table 7-28 highlights the differences.

Table 7-27. Model A and Model B: Service Profile (Residents) (percentages)

	1982		1981	
	Model B	Model A	Model B	Model A
Oral diagnosis	15.4	9.5	7.6	9.8
Prevention	2.4	1.1	4.4	2.9
Periodontics	9.2	7.7	4.7	4.5
Restorative without lab	28.3	19.1	33.6	16.8
Restorative with lab	12.7	23.1	15.0	20.4
Fixed prosthodontics	2.8	9.9	8.2	18.9
Removable prosthodontics	4.9	6.7	3.8	5.2
Endodontics	13.8	6.1	8.1	6.3
Orthodontics	0.4	1.7	1.2	1.7
Oral surgery	3.0	1.2	2.6	1.4
Other	7.2	14.1	11.1	12.3

Table 7-28. Model A and Model B: Chairside Hours Spent on Service Categories (Residents)

	Model B	Model A
Oral surgery	27	7
Endodontics	121	61
Periodontics	81	49
Diagnosis and prevention	156	67
Prosthodontics	67	105

SUMMARY
Model B residents generated more income, spent more time chairside, and emphasized more prevention, periodontics, and simple restorations than Model A residents, who emphasized crown and bridge procedures.

COMPARISONS BETWEEN STUDENTS IN MODELS A AND B
Because of the information-collection procedures used in the main dental school, it was impossible to compare Models A, B, and T students on the criteria given here. The clinical activity analysis (see Chapter 6) compares the three groups on all clinical activity variables for which information was available in Model T.

Seniors
In 1982, Model B seniors spent 29 percent more time at chairside, completed 40 percent more visits, and generated 44 percent more income than Model A seniors. In 1981, however, Model A seniors had more billable charges, more payments, and higher lab charges than Model B seniors (see Table 7-29).

Model A seniors spent 13 percent of their time on fixed prosthetics and 17 percent on removable prosthetics as compared to figures of 6 percent and 15 percent, respectively, for Model B seniors. Model B seniors spent relatively more time on periodontics: 9.2 percent (40 hours) and endodontics: 10.8 percent (47 hours) than Model A seniors: 6.9 percent on periodontics (23 hours) and 7.2 percent on endodontics (24 hours) (see Table 7-32).

Juniors
The two models are basically at the same level in this category. For chairside hours Model A juniors were 33 percent higher than Model B juniors. At the same time, however, Model B juniors completed 6 percent more visits. Payments to Model A juniors were 6 percent higher than payments to Model B juniors (see Table 7-30).

The relative time spent on various service categories followed the same pattern for the two groups, but in absolute numbers Model A juniors spent more time in almost every category of service (see Table 7-32).

Sophomores
Productive hours and number of visits were essentially the same for both groups of sophomores, but payments were twice as much for Model A sophomores (see Table 7-31). The main difference in the service profile is that Model A sophomores spent relatively more time on oral medicine (39 percent versus 27 percent) whereas Model B sophomores spent more time on periodontics (17 percent versus 34 percent) (see Table 7-32).

Table 7-29. Model A and Model B: Comparison of Student Productivity (Seniors)

	Fiscal Year	Productive Hours	Visits	Min./ Visit	Billable Charges	Payments	Lab Charges	Bill./ Visit	Lab/ Visit	Payment/ Visit
Model A	1982	337	197	103	8,673	8,193	1,524	44.09	7.75	41.75
	1981	463	266	104	15,338	9,192	4,118	57.59	15.46	34.51
Model B	1982	434	276	94	12,049	11,811	1,600	43.69	5.80	42.83
	1981	471	273	104	9,375	7,878	2,264	34.31	8.29	28.82

Table 7-30. Model A and Model B: Comparison of Student Productivity (Juniors)

	Fiscal Year	Productive Hours	Visits	Min./ Visit	Billable Charges	Payments	Lab Charges	Bill./ Visit	Lab/ Visit	Payment/ Visit
Model A	1982	426	199	128	6,487	6,203	412	32.60	2.07	31.17
	1981	372	213	105	6,604	4,043	159	30.95	.75	18.96
Model B	1982	320	211	91	8,059	5,832	473	38.51	2.29	27.87
	1981	381	209	109	5,090	4,055	463	24.32	2.21	19.40

Table 7-31. Model A and Model B: Comparison of Student Productivity (Sophomores)

	Fiscal Year	Productive Hours	Visits	Min./Visit	Billable Charges	Payments	Lab Charges	Bill./Visit	Lab/Visit	Payment/Visit
Model A	1982	28	12	139	243	199	–	20.00	–	9.85
	1981	50	24	125	407	366	7	12.25	.29	15.52
Model B	1982	24	10	142	125	99	–	12.20	–	9.66
	1981	17	7	146	291	156	–	43.15	–	23.15

Table 7-32. Model B: Comparison of Service Profiles

	Oral Diagnosis and Prevention		Perio-dontics		Operative		Prostho-dontics		Endo-dontics		Ortho-dontics		Oral Surgery		Other	
	82	81	82	81	82	81	82	81	82	81	82	81	82	81	82	81
Residents:																
Hours per person	155.5	79.8	80.5	31.6	357.8	319.7	66.8	100.0	120.8	71.8	3.3	5.9	26.5	11.1	63.0	46.2
%	17.8	12.0	9.2	4.7	40.9	48.6	7.6	15.4	13.8	10.8	0.3	1.1	3.0	3.4	7.2	4.1
Seniors:																
Hours per person	47.0	34.4	40.0	51.4	179.5	178.9	89.0	97.8	47.0	33.7	6.0	4.6	7.0	4.1	19.0	9.2
%	10.8	8.3	9.2	12.4	41.3	43.2	20.5	23.6	10.8	8.1	1.4	1.1	1.6	1.0	4.4	2.2
Juniors:																
Hours per person	66.0	37.6	35.0	57.5	138.5	186.6	33.5	18.8	32.5	40.0	0.0	3.6	5.5	7.4	7.0	3.7
%	20.8	10.6	11.0	16.2	43.6	52.6	10.5	5.3	10.2	11.3	0.0	1.0	1.7	2.1	2.2	1.0
Model total: *																
Hours	4,652	3,129	2,541	1,764	6,746	1,595	1,388	1,581	1,135	412	303	560	267	1,481	612	
%	23.8	22.0	13.0	12.4	34.5	38.3	8.2	10.3	8.1	2.1	2.3	2.9	2.0	7.6	4.5	
National average of dental practitioners (1982)	13.5%		4.6%		40.9%		23.0%		7.2%		2.2%		4.1%		4.2%	

* Includes faculty, hygienists, and sophomores.

Table 7-32. (continued).
Model A: Comparison of Service Profiles

	Oral Diagnosis and Prevention		Perio- dontics		Operative		Prostho- dontics		Endo- dontics		Ortho- dontics		Oral Surgery		Other	
	82	81	82	81	82	81	82	81	82	81	82	81	82	81	82	81
Residents:																
Hours per person	67.4	61.8	49.0	21.3	269.1	152.7	105.2	117.7	38.8	30.5	10.8	7.5	7.4	6.1	59.6	60.3
%	10.6	12.6	7.7	4.5	42.2	37.2	16.5	24.1	6.1	6.3	1.7	1.7	1.2	1.4	14.1	12.3
Seniors:																
Hours per person	29.3	38.1	23.3	35.6	140.0	188.5	100.7	117.2	15.4	33.8	2.1	1.6	7.4	3.0	9.9	10.5
%	8.7	8.9	6.9	8.3	41.5	44.0	29.9	27.4	7.2	7.9	0.6	0.4	2.9	0.7	3.4	2.5
Juniors:																
Hours per person	98.9	97.4	45.0	41.4	191.3	149.0	36.2	29.9	34.6	25.6	2.7	4.0	7.5	5.2	9.3	10.9
%	23.2	26.8	10.6	11.4	45.0	41.0	8.5	8.2	8.1	7.1	0.6	1.1	1.8	1.4	2.2	3.0
*Model total:**																
Hours	2,896	2,470	1,164	801	4,719	3,356	1,838	1,615	760	581	123	76	176	93	864	449
%	23.1	26.2	9.3	8.5	37.6	35.6	14.7	17.1	6.1	6.2	1.0	0.8	1.4	1.0	6.9	4.8
National Average of Dental Practitioners, 1982	13.5%		4.6%		40.9%		23.0%		7.2%		2.2%		4.1%		4.2%	

*Includes sophomores, hygiene residents, and hygiene students.

Management Dimension: Overall Summary

This section provides a detailed report of students' perceptions of the experimental work environment.

WORK ENVIRONMENT

One of the objectives of the experiment was to provide a work environment that complemented the innovative educational experience. Therefore, an important aspect of the managerial evaluation was the assessment and evaluation of students' perceptions of their work environments. This section includes extensive data comparing Models A, B, and T in this area, attempting to measure statistically the "quality of work life" in the experiment, which was, indeed, a significant feature of the Pennsylvania Experiment.

Methods and Samples

A questionnaire, the Work Environment Scale (WES), developed by P. M. Insel and R. H. Moos,[2] was selected to determine the main characteristics of the work environment in the different programs of the dental school, thereby determining whether there were any significant differences between the environments of Models A, B, and T (and also detecting any changes that occurred between FY81 and FY82 as a result of the interactive planning effort).

The questionnaire consists of ninety true-false statements about different aspects of the work environment. It is organized around ten dimensions: involvement, peer cohesion, staff support, autonomy, task orientation, work pressure, clarity, control, innovation, and physical comfort (see Table 7-33). The scores of each respondent were standardized according to a conversion table, in which 50 represents the mean value, with a standard deviation of 10. This adjustment makes the data of every dimension comparable in scale.

Statements that were felt by the student to be not applicable were not considered, and scores were adjusted accordingly. During the two-year period of the analysis, more than twenty samples were taken from the following groups: dental students, dental hygiene students, faculty, residents, and staff.

In each of the clinical settings (Models A, B, and T) a sample of students from each class during 1981 and 1982 completed the WES in April or May. In addition, in December 1981, juniors and seniors from the traditional program were asked to complete the WES to determine whether there were any differences among different instructional groups. (The traditional program divides all seniors and juniors into ten instructional groups in which the students complete nearly all their restorative and periodontal clinical education.) Of the ten instructional groups, four were sampled and completed the WES. Only one sample of dental hygiene students was taken in 1981. In 1981, samples of the

Table 7-33. Work Environment Scale-Subscale Description

Dimension		Relationship Dimensions
1.	Involvement	Measures the extent to which workers are concerned about and committed to their jobs; includes terms designed to reflect enthusiasm and constructive activity.
2.	Peer cohesion	Measures the extent to which workers are friendly to and supportive of each other.
3.	Staff support	Measures the extent to which management is supportive of workers and encourages workers to be supportive of each other.
		Personal Growth Dimensions
4.	Autonomy	Assesses the extent to which workers are encouraged to be self-sufficient and to make their own decisions. Includes items related to personal development and growth.
5.	Task orientation	Assesses the extent to which the climate emphasizes good planning and efficiency and encourages workers to "get the job done."
		System-Maintenance and System Change Dimensions
6.	Work pressure	Measures the extent to which the pressure of work dominates the job milieu.
7.	Clarity	Measures the extent to which workers know what to expect in their daily routines and how explicitly rules and policies are communicated.
8.	Control	Measures the extent to which management uses rules and pressures to keep workers under control.
9.	Innovation	Measures the extent to which variety, change, and new approaches are emphasized in the work environment.
10.	Physical comfort	Assesses the extent to which the physical surroundings contribute to a pleasant work environment.

faculty, residents, students, and staff of Model A and of Model B were taken. The 1981 results are presented in Figure 7-3.

Analysis

In 1981, the WES results for third- and fourth-year dental students, residents, staff, and faculty were similar. Because of personnel changes, sample sizes, and the logistics of administration, the WES was administered only to dental students during the second year of the evaluation, 1981–82. This procedure allowed measures of the A, B, and T programs to be taken at both the clinical and preclinical stages. The dental student samples were organized in the following way: Model A and B programs were combined during the preclinical years and compared to T (since the preclinical programs are the same for stu-

Figure 7-3. Work Environment Scale, Models A and B, 1981

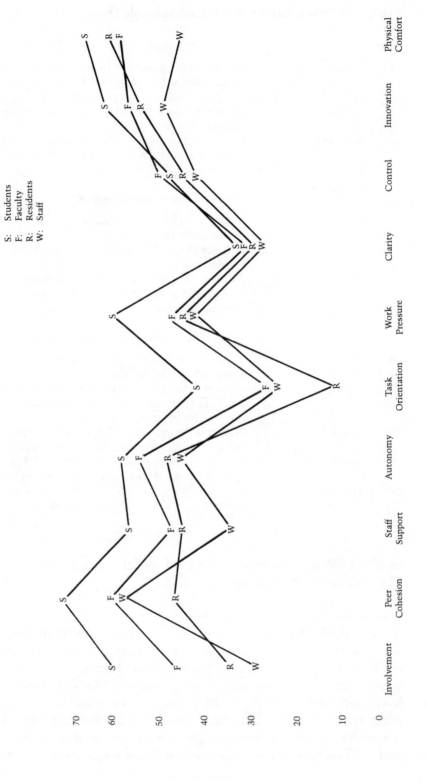

S: Students
F: Faculty
R: Residents
W: Staff

dents from both experimental models), and for the last two years, responses of students from A, B, and T were compared separately.

In summary, ten samples were collected. The sample sizes are shown in Table 7-34.

Figures 7-4 through 7-5 illustrate the mean value for each dimension of the instrument, according to the respondent group. Each figure presents the data of two groups at a time, to enhance the comparison of related groups. In Figures 7-4 through 7-8, the changes of each group from 1981 to 1982 are seen (T preclinical, T clinical, A and B preclinical, B clinical, A clinical), while Figures 7-9 through 7-16 represent the differences and similarities of the different programs (T versus A and so on).

Results

The preclinical years of the traditional program (Figure 7-4) showed statistically significant changes from 1981 to 1982 in the areas of student environment, task orientation, clarity of directions, and comfort. They were all positive changes, indicating a general improvement in the work environment. There were no significant changes for the two clinical years in Model T in any area (Figure 7-5).

The preclinical years for Models A and B (Figure 7-6) do not show significant changes between 1981 and 1982, except in innovation. Students perceived the environment as less innovative in 1982 than in 1981.

No statistical change was detected in the clinical work environment of Model B between 1981 and 1982 (Figure 7-7). In 1982, the clinical work environment in Model A (Figure 7-8) improved significantly in task orientation. Although not significant at the $p < .01$ level, this program also showed important improvements in 1982 in the areas of involvement, peer cohesion, staff support, autonomy, clarity, and work pressure, reflecting a possible general improvement and a higher level of activity. A significant decrease in physical comfort was felt in Model A (Figure 7-8), perhaps reflecting an increase in numbers of students in the program in 1981–82, which increased chair demand.

Figures 7-9 and 7-10 compare the work environment profiles of the traditional and experimental programs (A and B combined) in the two preclinical

Table 7-34. Sample Size of Dental Student Groups Completing Work Environmental Scale

Year	Preclinical		Clinical		
	T	*A and B*	*T*	*A*	*B*
1981	101	21	10	10	8
1982	191	18	21	15	8

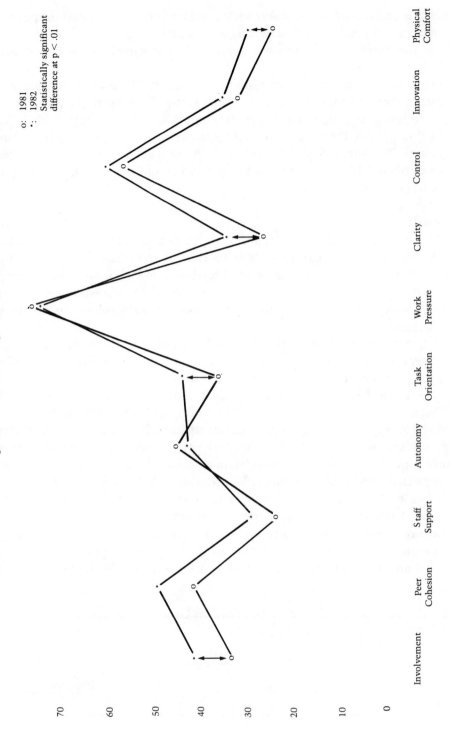

Figure 7-4. Traditional Program, Preclinical Years 1981–1982

o: 1981
•: 1982
Statistically significant
difference at p < .01

Involvement Peer Cohesion Staff Support Autonomy Task Orientation Work Pressure Clarity Control Innovation Physical Comfort

0 10 20 30 40 50 60 70

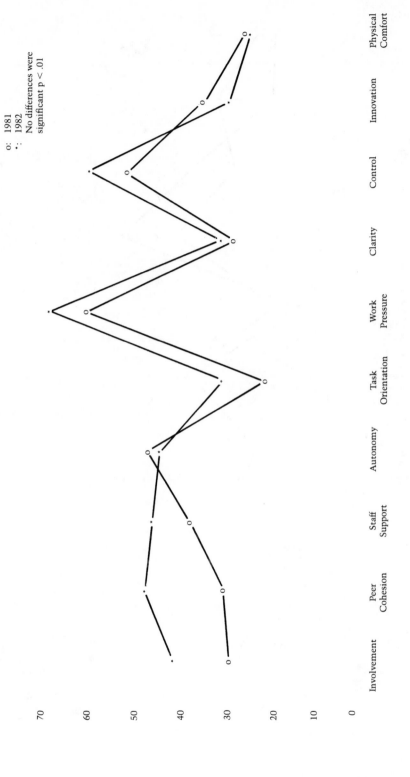

Figure 7-5. Traditional Program, Clinical Years

o: 1981
•: 1982
No differences were
significant p < .01

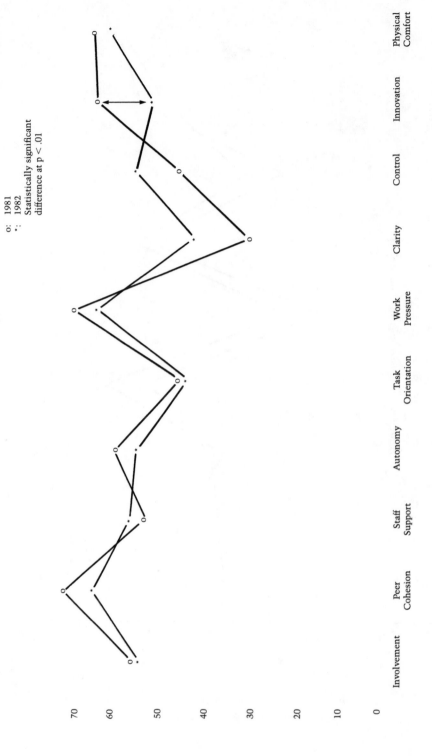

Figure 7-6. Experimental Program A and B Combined, Preclinical Years

o: 1981
·: 1982
Statistically significant
difference at p < .01

Figure 7-7. Experimental Program Model B, Clinical Years 1981–1982

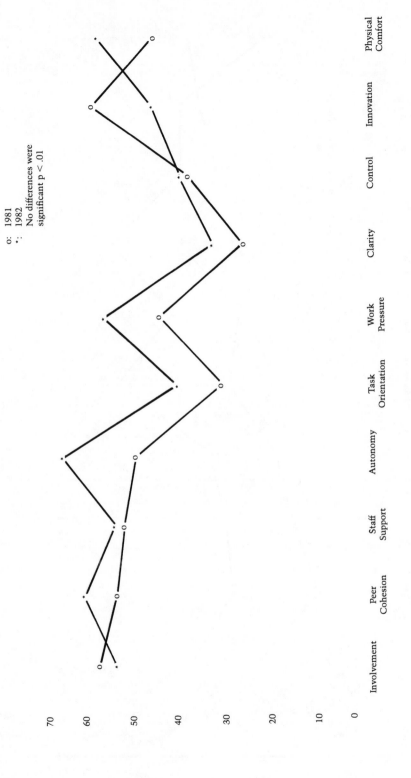

o: 1981
*: 1982
No differences were
significant p < .01

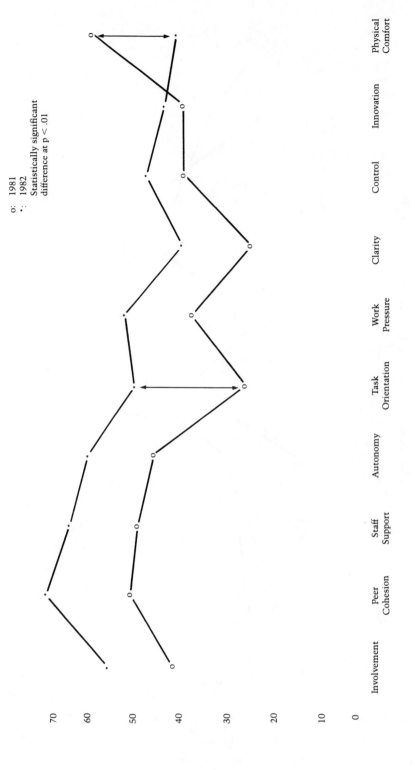

Figure 7-8. Experimental Program Model A, Clinical Years 1981–1982

o: 1981
*: 1982
Statistically significant
difference at p < .01

Involvement   Peer   Staff   Autonomy   Task   Work   Clarity   Control   Innovation   Physical
              Cohesion Support   Orientation Pressure   Comfort

Figure 7-9. Traditional Program versus Experimental Programs (A and B Combined), Preclinical Year 1981

o: Model T
*: Models A and B
Statistically significant difference at p < .01

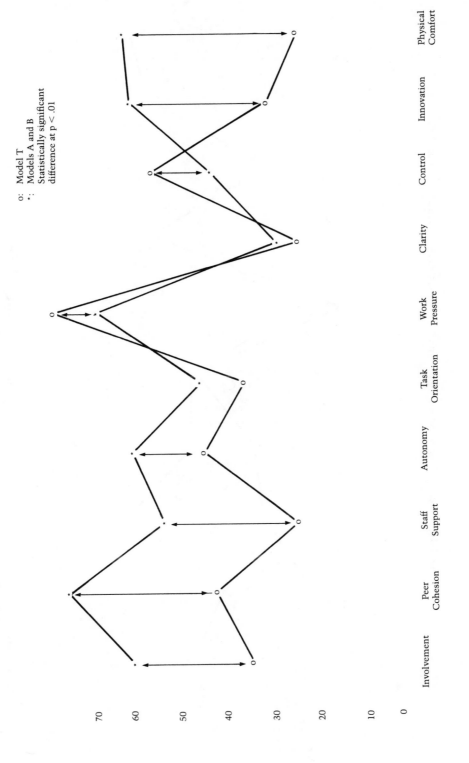

Figure 7-10. Traditional Program versus Experimental Programs (A and B Combined), Preclinical Year 1982

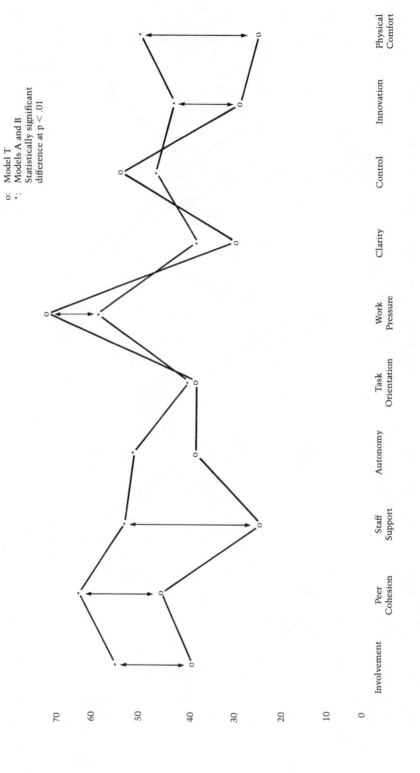

o: Model T
*: Models A and B
Statistically significant
difference at p < .01

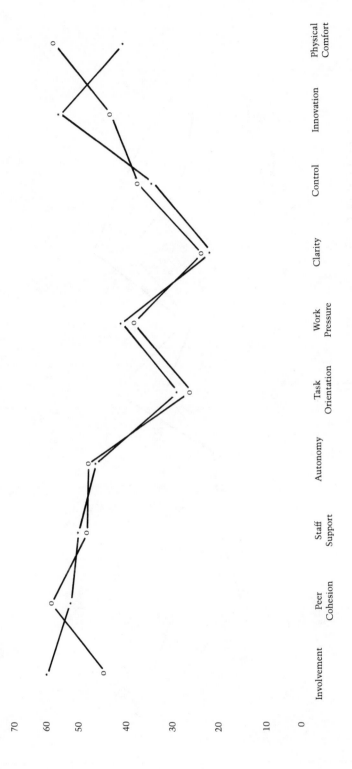

Figure 7-11. Experimental Program A versus Experimental Program B, Clinical Year 1981

o: Model A
·: Model B
No differences were significant p < .01

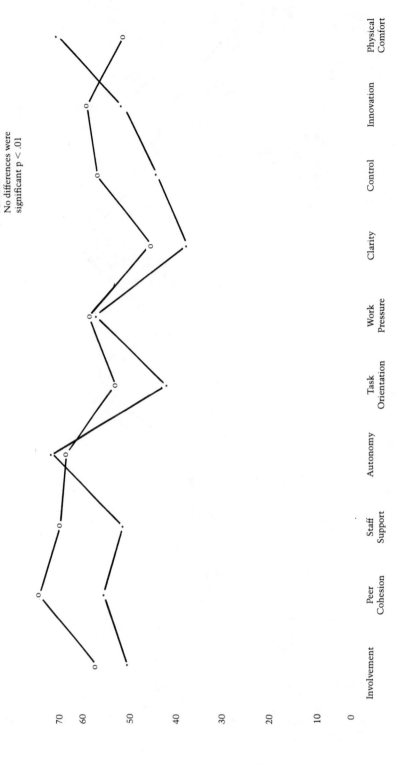

Figure 7-12. Experimental Program A versus Experimental Program B, Clinical Year 1982

o: Model A
•: Model B
No differences were
significant p < .01

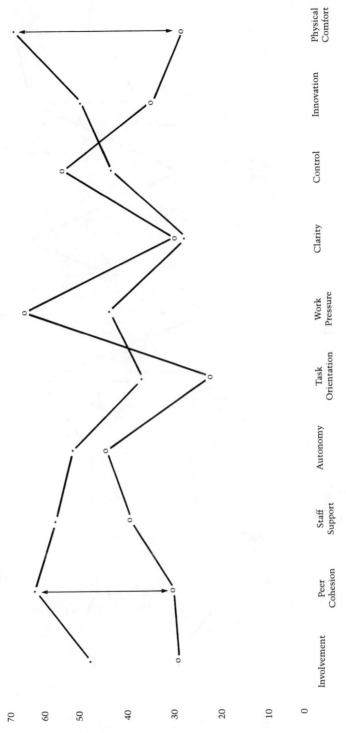

Figure 7-13. Traditional Program versus Experimental Program A, Clinical Year 1981

o: Model T
•: Model A
Statistically significant
difference at p < .01

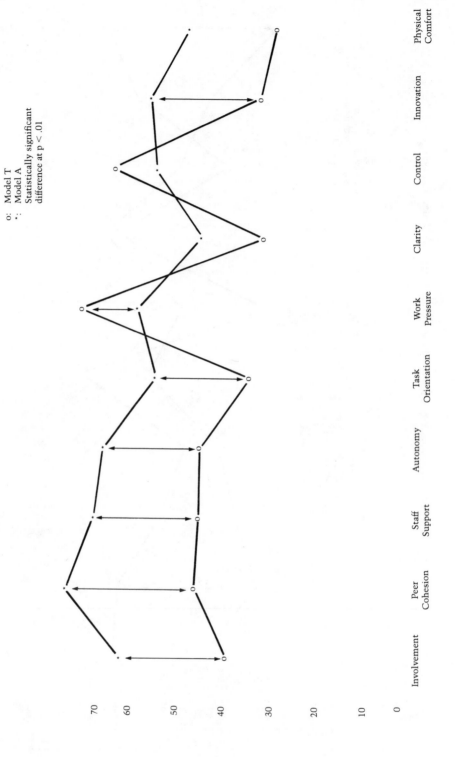

Figure 7-14. Traditional Program versus Experimental Program A, Clinical Year 1982

o: Model T
•: Model A
Statistically significant
difference at p < .01

Figure 7-15. Traditional Program versus Experimental Program B, Clinical Year 1981

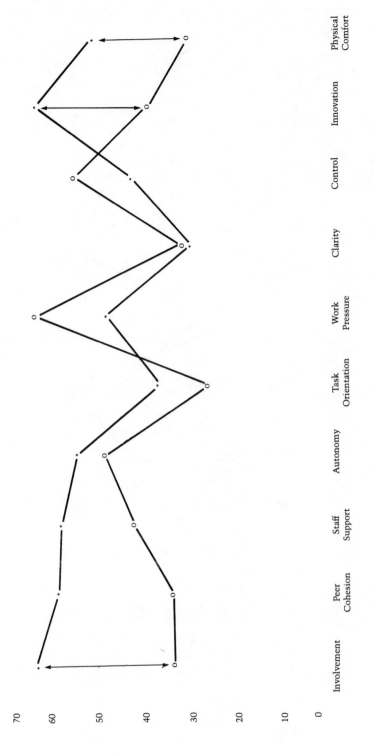

o: Model T
*: Model B
Statistically significant difference at p < .01

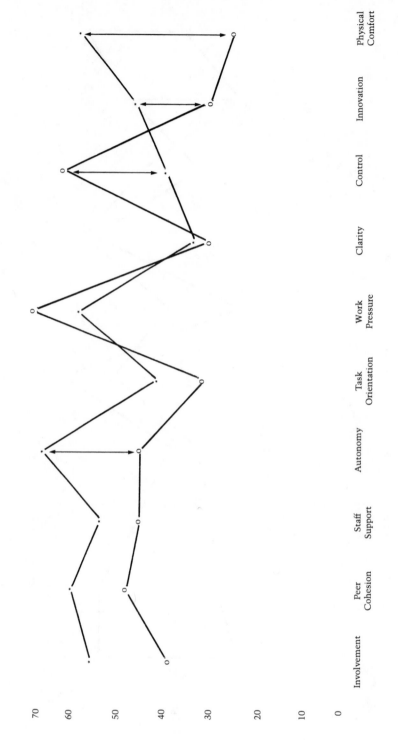

Figure 7-16. Traditional Program versus Experimental Program B, Clinical Year 1982

o: Model T
•: Model B
Statistically significant
difference at p < .01

years for 1981 and 1982. There are many significant differences (p < .01) between these programs in the preclinical years. Programs A and B have higher levels of involvement, peer cohesion, staff support, innovation, and comfort for both years, and of autonomy and control in 1982. Work pressure and control are significantly lower in the new programs. These results suggest a better work environment in the experimental preclinical program than in the traditional preclinical program.

As Figures 7-11 and 7-12 demonstrate, there are no significant differences in the clinical years between Model A and Model B. Physical comfort seemed to have decreased in Model A from 1981 to 1982, but in other areas a general improvement of Model A over Model B can be detected.

Comparing the traditional program and Model A over the two years demonstrates that in 1982, A received significantly better ratings than the traditional program in most areas of the WES (Figures 7-13 and 7-14). Comparing the clinical years of Models T and B (Figures 7-15 and 7-16) shows similar results. Model B's work environment is generally perceived as superior to that of the traditional program.

The following conclusions can be made from these data: In the preclinical years, the experimental program is rated significantly higher in most areas of the Work Environment Scale than the traditional program. The clinical years in Models A and B are also perceived as superior to the clinical years in T although the differences are not as pronounced as for the preclinical years. Differences between the models themselves in the clinical years are insignificant; they are perceived similarly as work environments.

These results suggest that the experimental work environment is perceived differently than the traditional work environment. In particular, for both 1981 and 1982, in the preclinical years, involvement, peer cohesion, staff support, work pressure, innovation, and physical comfort were significantly better in the experimental work environment than in the traditional work environment. For the 1982 clinical year, Model A's work environment was perceived as superior to that of the traditional program. Also, the students perceived Model B's work environment as better than the traditional work environment, although the differences were not as pronounced as those between Model A and the traditional program. In summary, the experimental environments seem to foster a better work climate than the traditional program. This information is consistent with open-ended interviews conducted by members of the Busch Center (see Chapter 8), in which students consistently stated that they preferred the experimental program.

One possible confounding variable in this analysis is the question of whether educational differences account for the difference in students' perceptions of the work environment. In part to address this possibility, student evaluations of instructors in the traditional and experimental programs were collected and compared. The average overall ratings of teaching in courses in each program in the school in 1980–81 and 1981–82 are summarized in Tables 7-35 and 7-36. (Five is the highest rating and one is the lowest.)

Table 7-35. Lecture Instructor Evaluations

	1980–81		1981–82	
	Mean	St. Dev.	Mean	St. Dev.
Clinical science (trad.)	3.84	1.06	4.15	2.70
Basic science (trad.)	3.84	1.06	3.86	1.10
Pennsylvania Experiment	4.26	.98	3.96	1.14
Dental hygiene	4.36	.82	4.38	.83
All departments (trad.)	3.92	1.03	4.08	1.67

Table 7-36. Clinic/Lab Instructor Evaluations

	1980–81		1981–82	
	Mean	St. Dev.	Mean	St. Dev.
Clinical science (trad.)	4.10	1.04	4.13	1.01
Basic science (trad.)	4.07	.98	4.30	.94
Pennsylvania Experiment	4.52	.77	4.49	.83
Dental hygiene	4.56	.74	4.59	.74
All departments (trad.)	4.21	.97	4.24	.95

The mean overall evaluation of instructors is not significantly different among programs ($p < .01$). Therefore, a difference in the perceived quality of teaching does not seem to be a factor in explaining the observed differences in the work environments.

Discussion

Most institutions try to create environments that will facilitate the achievement of their goals or maximize growth in certain areas. It cannot be stated conclusively that an improved work environment in the dental school leads to better dentists, but it is likely that a high-quality work environment contributes significantly to the fulfillment of the school's goals in the areas of education and finance.

Given the above information, it appears that the experimental work environments are different from the traditional work environment. This is expected since the experimental environment was created as an innovative and differentiated experience. As part of this experimental environment, clerical support systems were made available to students, decision-making autonomy was achieved by students, peer and supervisor interaction were encouraged, required cases were more readily available, and the physical environment was designed for the comfort of the patients and the individuals treating the patients.

It appears that the experiment does indeed provide an improved work environment, which, theoretically, has enhanced the students' learning process and has relieved many of the stresses often associated with dental school.

Notes

1. James F. Galbally and Cecile A. Feldman, "University of Pennsylvania School of Dental Medicine Financial Planning Simulation," *Penn Dental Journal* 84, no. 2 (1982): 13–17.
2. P. M. Insel and R. H. Moos, *Work Environment Scale* (Consulting Psychologists Press, California, 1974).

8

Summary and Conclusions

This chapter summarizes and discusses the results of the experiment, based on the findings of the Busch Center and the experiences of the authors as codirectors of the Pennsylvania Experiment. The chapter begins with a discussion of student interviews conducted by the Busch Center and faculty interviews conducted by the authors.

Student and Faculty Interviews

As the Busch Center noted, the purpose of evaluation is to determine whether an experiment worked, based on a specific set of educational tests and measures. Yet much of the essence of an experiment involves the day-to-day experiences of the people who are involved in it—the feelings, opinions, and subjective impressions of students, faculty, and administrators. These impressions are often difficult to categorize as indicators of "success" or "failure," but they nevertheless add an important dimension to any discussion of the overall effects of an experiment.

For this reason, the Busch Center conducted open-ended interviews with students involved in the Pennsylvania Experiment to capture their impressions of some of the subjective aspects of the program. Selections from these interviews are included here, as well as selections from open-ended interviews conducted with the principal members of the faculty and administration.

Student volunteers from both experimental models and from the traditional program were solicited for interviews concerning their reactions to the experiment. Twelve students from the experiment volunteered; however, no students in the traditional program offered to be interviewed. Thus the interviews have a built-in bias in that those who did not volunteer were not interviewed.

Perhaps the single aspect of the experiment that was discussed most consistently by students was their perception that the quality of life in the new program was an improvement over that of the traditional program. All twelve students interviewed indicated that, given a choice, they would again select the Pennsylvania Experiment over the traditional program. This finding was indicated to some extent by the Work Environment Scale (see Chapter 7); these interviews strongly corroborate the findings of that measure.

All of the twelve students interviewed made some reference to improved quality of life, reporting that relationships, working conditions, and other aspects were much less stressful in the experiment than in the traditional program. Many reasons for this perceived improvement were offered, including better student-faculty ratios, improved facilities, and a spirit of idealism that accompanied the new program. Although it is difficult to determine the relative importance of each of these factors, it is clear that at least some of the students in the experiment (those who agreed to be interviewed) perceived a marked difference in the quality of life.

Some typical responses follow:

Senior, Model B: "I think the positive things about being here have been the modern facilities, the personal relationships with the auxiliaries, dentists, and classmates. The fact that the instructors get to know you . . . there is less stress, I think you can just generally do more work here for all the reasons that there is less red tape and you can just do more clinical work rather than spend your time in lines. Most of my friends hated dental school because of the hassles they thought they've had all through those school years. I don't feel that way at all; I've enjoyed dental school; I thought it was great."

Senior, Model B: "The environment that we work in is far superior to the dental school. The ease of getting materials and equipment and the working conditions themselves are far more conducive to a more pleasant experience than Model T. Not having to wait in lines for things, less paperwork, make things a lot more pleasant. . . . It was a very positive experience."

Senior, Model A: In response to the question, "Is there any particular area that you thought was especially good about this program as opposed to the traditional program?"

"There are hundreds of things . . . a lot of the advantages were simply the overall ambience of the situation down there; the closeness that people have with each other, the faculty and the students. . . . I think the things that you can't deny are that the student-faculty ratio is better, that you get to know people on a much more personal basis, and that the clinic is just much more pleasant. You never feel as though you're fighting against anyone. You never have anybody say anything negative to you unless it is done tactfully or with a smile or something like that. I think that's a definite advantage."

Although students interviewed were unanimous in preferring the experimental environment, they also mentioned areas that were stressful and less than optimal. Each student listed approximately two to three disadvantages in the work environment of the experiment. Areas mentioned by more than one student included lack of clear communications between administration, faculty, and students; and lack of information about the overall operation of the models.

A majority of the students interviewed also felt that the Pennsylvania Experiment offered a superior education. Nine of the twelve felt that they had received a superior education; the remaining three felt that it was at least equivalent.

In interviews with the principal faculty members and administrators, similar responses emerged. Both directors of the models claimed that students in their programs were receiving a superior education when compared with the education received by students in other programs with which they were involved. The director of Model B expressed the belief that students in his program were far ahead of students at equivalent stages whom he had taught in the traditional program. These principals also felt that the results of the Busch Report did not fully reflect the value of the experiment and that the report captured only a limited perspective of the educational differences offered by the new program. Faculty members also noticed strong differences in the attitudes of students in the experiment: their overall demeanor was one of enthusiasm and excitement about their education, and the passivity and apathy sometimes associated with dental school seemed to be missing. Thus, according to these interviews, the experiment appears to have had a strong impact in the more subjective but nevertheless important areas of quality of life within a dental school.

Summary and Conclusions

SUMMARY OF EDUCATIONAL RESULTS

In reviewing the findings of the Busch Center, certain results are clear-cut. Educationally, the Pennsylvania Experiment produced students with at least comparable psychomotor skills to those in the traditional program at the University of Pennsylvania. These skills include basic preclinical and clinical tasks. Further, the cognitive skills of these students, as measured by grade point average and National Boards and Northeast Regional Boards, are also equivalent.

At the same time, these students are, according to the data, engaging in more clinical activity. They are performing these procedures in a mix that closely resembles the ideal of the highly competent generalist—concentrating less on restorative procedures and more on areas that will be central to the generalist practice of the future: periodontics and prevention. The junior and senior treatment-planning examinations indicate that experimental students have attained basic levels of treatment planning comparable to those attained by students within the traditional program.

It may be that the strongest differences between the traditional and experi-

mental programs lie in the less quantifiable but equally important area of affective education. The patient situation test revealed significant differences in
student responses to patients, with those educated within the experiment re-
vealing consistently more understanding responses. This finding may reflect
the success of the human behavior course; however, it may also be a by-product
of educating students within a smaller, more humane environment—one that
provides faculty role models demonstrating sophisticated interpersonal skills.
The dental hygiene questionnaire also revealed that students in the experiment developed more respect for and knowledge about the role of the dental
hygienist, presumably through the integration of hygienists into their clinical
education. These affective aspects of the students' education—changes in attitude toward the hygienist and more effective interpersonal skills—combined
with students' increased performance of those functions traditionally associated with the specialist indicate that, to some extent, the Pennsylvania Experiment succeeded in educating a more competent generalist than did the
traditional program. There is, however, no evidence in the data that these students are better prepared to perform treatment planning for their patients than
are traditional students. Nevertheless, in several key areas, students in the experiment appear to be better prepared to act as competent generalists.

Students and faculty alike expressed a high degree of enthusiasm about their
educational experiences within the experiment. Although these attitudes have
not been quantified and cannot be presented as hard data, it does appear from
subjective impressions that the problem of "quality of life" within dental
school was successfully addressed by the experiment. In an era of decreased
enrollments for dental schools, this aspect of the experiment is particularly
relevant. Unlike many dental students, student participants in the models did
not dislike their dental school experience; on the contrary, they often liked it
enough to select their experimental models as the site of their future professional practices and teaching careers. This may be one facet of the solution to
the growing problems of recruitment and enrollment of students.

The limitations of the Busch Report must also be repeated here. The experiment was a new program of education that was being tested for its financial
and educational viability. Therefore, the questions asked by the evaluation
were pragmatic ones: Is this program financially viable? Does it educate students at least comparably to the traditional program? It is possible to ask any
number of other questions of the Pennsylvania Experiment; the richness and
complexity of the program were very difficult to capture by the data revealed
in the Busch Center report. Also, the report was based on two years of data
collection, which can be viewed only as preliminary information on the overall
effects of the new program. Thus it can best be viewed as a snapshot taken
from a particular angle at a fixed point in time.

Perhaps one of the most important questions which is as yet unexplored is
that of the career development of students educated in the experiment. The
question of whether the Pennsylvania Experiment prepares students to func-

tion as highly competent generalists was, to some extent, answered by the Busch Report. The manner in which these skills will actually be used by students in their careers, however, remains to be seen. The effects of previous innovative programs implemented at the School of Dental Medicine on students were not apparent until five, ten, and sometimes twenty years after the student had graduated. In the Periodontal Prothesis Program, for example, a very high percentage of graduates went on to distinguish themselves in careers in dental research, education, and practice. This dimension of an educational study can be measured only by a longitudinal study, which is, of course, impossible at this time. Thus the long-term effects and ramifications of the experiment remain unknown. Some early signs that students reared in the experiment may manifest unusual career patterns are already present; for example, a high percentage of the students in the experiment have remained at the school, often teaching and practicing in the models. Also, many students educated in the experiment have pursued careers in postgraduate work or in hospital or public health settings. It is certain that the educational effects of the experiment will become clearer and more apparent with the passage of time.

SUMMARY OF FINANCIAL AND MANAGERIAL RESULTS

Perhaps one of the most promising results in the financial area was the success of the residency program. Residents educated in Models A and B were more productive than the national average for residency programs, and the overall residency program achieved financial viability. These findings indicate particularly promising results.

Model B

As the Busch Center noted, the Pennsylvania Experiment also demonstrated that a financially viable, faculty-based practice-educational unit is possible. Model B demonstrated that such practices can be financially self-sustaining and can serve as potential sources of added income to a dental school. The Model B facility also provided many valuable lessons on the criteria for successful practice-educational units. These lessons are presented here so that institutions and educators desiring to implement similar programs can benefit from the experiences at Pennsylvania.

The role of the clinician-educator was the crux of the new program. As the experiment progressed, it became apparent that, to a great extent, the clinician-educator determines the success or failure of such a program. As the preceptor, he/she is at the heart of the new model. In starting a Model B type facility, *it is critically important to identify qualified clinician-educators.* Unfortunately, the experiment also indicated that it is very difficult to accomplish this; to date, very few such individuals exist within dental education.

Accordingly, the experiment witnessed a very high clinician-educator turnover rate. Several high-quality dentists found the position to be unsuitable for their personal styles and preferences. The position requires a faculty member who can practice under the highest standards and at the same time provide students with constant direction and guidance. He/she also must be willing, to some extent, to sacrifice the autonomy and open-ended financial incentives traditionally associated with dental practice. The position is not suitable for a dentist who is merely looking for a diversion from teaching or practice; rather, it is for someone who wants to perform both roles more fully.

The best way to identify successful clinician-educators may be to rear them within the faculty-practice system. In this way, practitioners have a good working knowledge of preceptorship, as well as a commitment to making the practice work. Of course, this is a long-term solution. It may be necessary to begin a few Model B practices on a very small scale, gradually phasing in more practitioners as they become available. It is also important to give the clinician-educator healthy financial incentives and guarantees of career security through devices such as the clinician-educator track.

In establishing a faculty practice it is useful, whenever possible, to bring in practitioners who already have an adequate patient base. What is perhaps most essential is that aggressive marketing efforts be launched to support the new practices; third-party programs involving institutions affiliated with the dental school are particularly promising for building a patient base.

The clinician-educator must have a fair degree of autonomy in managing his/her practice. These practitioners must meet the standards of the dental school, but they should have the freedom to manage their practices independently; it is probably unrealistic to expect a master clinician to function effectively without this freedom. To retain strict administrative control over such practices may be self-defeating.

Also, it is important to realize that a Model B-type practice requires a large population base to support the education of relatively small numbers of students. Third-party programs involving institutions are probably the most practical solution to the problem of securing a sufficient patient base. This becomes particularly relevant as an atmosphere of competitiveness and oversupply continues to grow within the dental profession. Dental professionals are likely to view Model B-type practices as unwelcome competition in an already stressful marketplace. It may therefore be preferable to implement one or two Model B's rather than a group of Model B's, given current realities within the professional environment.

Model A

In contrast to Model B, Model A, the Paletz Clinic, did not attain financial viability during its three years of operation. The Busch Report noted several of the key areas that required modification so that this viability could be attained. In general, it appears that in a larger clinical setting such as Model A, many of the amenities of the Model B private practice could not be retained. For example, exercising no control over the allocation of student supplies was not financially viable in Model A.

Another lesson provided by both models is that whether one is discussing a Model A or a Model B setting, it is essential that both faculty and students are educated about the overall operation of the facility. Foremost is the area of collections: it is all too easy for members of an educational unit to overlook collecting payment for services; however, such collection is obviously essential if the unit is to survive. Interestingly, faculty members with years of private practice experience tended to neglect this important area, presumably because they were in an educational environment. Also, treating both faculty and students as active, responsible members of the practice is essential; the single negative response cited most frequently in student interviews was a lack of knowledge about the overall working of the models. In implementing a program such as the Pennsylvania Experiment, the managerial structure should support the innovative nature of the program, including faculty, students, and staff, in organizational decision making.

The Pennsylvania Experiment also demonstrated that it is difficult to start a school within a school. Such a venture creates an entirely different set of problems than those normally associated with a new program. Faculty members within the traditional program naturally feel threatened by a change that affects the entire education of a significant group of students. If a school within a school is developed, it is critical that faculty and students outside of the new program be educated about the program and supported within their own structure. These efforts will, it is hoped, minimize any feelings of lack of control or competitiveness among members of the traditional program. It may be preferable to implement a new model such as this in a new school rather than trying to superimpose it on a program that has functioned differently for a substantial period of time.

The experiment repeatedly demonstrated another phenomenon: large-scale educational ventures such as this require flexibility and often compromise within the experimental design. Models A and B existed within a dynamic, complex professional and educational environment—one that constantly molded and reshaped their direction. Many times, it was necessary to sacrifice what might have been more desirable from a purely experimental point of view in order to meet the requirements of the university and the dental school. Many adjustments also had to be made so as not to compromise the students' education. If a particular program or approach was not working, it had to be changed. The authors strongly recommend the reflection-in-action model described in Chapter 4 as a useful tool for viewing this type of educational experiment. It is apparent that traditional models of social experimentation are not viable in situations such as this one.

Finally, an evaluation of the Pennsylvania Experiment would not be complete without acknowledging the goals that were not accomplished and that remain to be considered for future educational programs. In spite of several attempts by the experiment administration, the implementation of an oral biology track was not accomplished during the course of the experiment. This option is currently being examined.

Although the Pennsylvania Experiment succeeded in many ways in educating the "dentist of the future," in some areas this goal remains to be realized. In defining the dentist of the future, the original designers of the experiment stated: "The dental professional who will best be prepared for the future and who will best serve the population will be that person who . . . possesses a broad understanding of his/her role in society." This aspect of the dentist of the future was only partially developed in the experiment. Future programs should educate the dentist who thinks of the needs of the population as a whole rather than addressing only the needs of the patient as an individual. Issues such as reducing barriers to care and planning for the overall needs of the population were touched upon minimally in the new curriculum.

The Pennsylvania Experiment did succeed in educating dental students with a generalist orientation, prepared to assume many of the tasks traditionally delegated to the specialist, within an improved educational environment that used faculty talents more fully. Further, it created a model that made progress in improving quality of life within dental school and in addressing many of the pressing concerns in dental education today. It produced a financially successful faculty-based practice/educational unit and a self-sustaining fifth-year residency program. Many of the innovative trends that have appeared in dental education during the past twenty years were incorporated into the experiment, and many of the flaws traditionally associated with it (such as lack of integration between preclinical and clinical courses, fragmented clinical education, overcrowding and poor student-faculty ratios) were eliminated. The experiment clearly made great strides in demonstrating the possibilities that exist within dental education even during troubled economic times. These possibilities offer potential direction and solutions to institutions of dental education in an era of crisis and challenge.

Epilogue: The Pennsylvania Experiment Becomes the Pennsylvania Plan

The Pennsylvania Experiment ended officially at the close of academic year 1981–82. Many of the innovations and concepts that it represents have continued to develop at the School of Dental Medicine and are now integral components of the overall academic program at Pennsylvania.

In January 1983, Dean Designate Jan Lindhe stated to the Faculty Senate that the Pennsylvania Experiment is now the "Pennsylvania Plan." Since that time, efforts have been made to convert the experiment into a workable model for the entire dental school. The resulting program is based on the Model A system of education, with modifications to improve financial viability according to the lessons of the experiment. For example, students no longer have unlimited access to supplies as they did during the experiment; stricter control over the requisitioning of supplies are now in effect. Another major change is that rotations are now part of the modified Model A curriculum. Nevertheless, students still witness specialty procedures being performed in the integrated, generalist Model A setting. Thus, although, for example, they can perform oral surgery within the Model A clinic, they also rotate to the oral surgery department. Preclinical learning still takes place directly adjacent to the clinical setting, and students remain in one group throughout their four years of dental school.

Based on these modifications, the school opened its first modified Model A facility in 1983–84. Plans for the construction of several other Model A facilities are currently under way. In 1983–84, all first-year students and twenty students from each of the second-, third-, and fourth-year classes were being educated in either the new Model A or the original Model B. Plans call for the incorporation of all dental students into either a Model A setting or the Model B site by 1985–86.

Although Model B continues to function as a financially successful private practice/educational unit, plans to construct more facilities based on this model are not currently in effect primarily because of a perception of an oversupply of dental professionals. Although Model B is financially self-sufficient,

183

a relatively small number of students can be educated within this setting, compared to the large patient base required to make it financially viable. Another major barrier to constructing more Model B's at this time is the difficulty of identifying sufficient master clinicians qualified to direct such facilities. Accordingly, Model B remains as an example of the potential for the future and continues to educate approximately sixteen students per year as well as serving as a clinical laboratory for continuous educational experimentation.

Another creation of the Pennsylvania Experiment, the development of the fifth-year program in general dentistry, received full accreditation in November 1983 as one of the nation's first advanced general dentistry programs that is nonhospital based. It continues to flourish within the modified Model A and the Model B settings.

In December 1983, Dean Lindhe reaffirmed the school's commitment to the lessons and precepts of the Pennsylvania Experiment, stating that the modified Model A is now the D.M.D. curriculum and that Model B is the "learning laboratory" for the School of Dental Medicine.

Recognition of the Pennsylvania Experiment has begun to spread to other members of the dental education community as well. In a publication discussing outpatient clinics in the 1990s, Dr. Harry Bohannon stated that "Bob Tisot's Model B clinic at the University of Pennsylvania is a forerunner of tomorrow's dental school clinic."[1] It is hoped that the information contained in this book will stimulate this interest and will provide useful material to other members of the dental education community interested in pursuing similar innovative programs in their own schools. The experiment demonstrated many exciting possibilities for dental education; how these plans are built upon in the future lies in the ability of dental education to engage in new directions for the education of a dentist.

Note

1. Harry M. Bohannon, "Operating Outpatient Clinics in 1990," *Journal of Dental Education* 48, no. 6 (1984): 54.

Appendixes

APPENDIX I

Members of the First Long Range Planning Committee

D. Walter Cohen
Daniel Dhody
Arthur Freedman
James Galbally
Philip Graitcer

William Hickey
Howard Myers
Jay Seibert
Anthony Vito
John Yancey

APPENDIX II

Members of the Task Force on the Academic Future of the School of Dental Medicine

James Ackerman
John Amsterdam
Tom Backenstose
D. Walter Cohen
Patricia Cormier
Daniel Dhody
James Galbally
Benjamin Hammond

Daniel Isaacson
Charles Jerge
Samuel Martin
Howard Myers
Joel Rosenbloom
Jay Seibert
Irwin Ship

APPENDIX III

Members of the Second Long Range Planning Committee

James Ackerman
John Amsterdam
Morton Amsterdam

Howard Myers
Maurice Perreault
Mark Portnoy

Robert Beideman
Vernon Brightman
Pamela Brown
D. Walter Cohen
Robert DeRevere
James Galbally
John Hellwege
Charles Jerge
Malcolm Lynch
Daniel McCollum

Joel Rosenbloom
Michele Saunders
Jay Seibert
Irwin Ship
Robert Vanarsdall
Anthony Vito
Dale Wade
Irene Woodall
Stephen Wotman
Robert Zemsky

APPENDIX IV

National Advisory Board

Howard Bailit
Professor and Chairman
Department of Health Administration
Columbia University
School of Public Health
600 West 168th Street
New York, NY 10032

David Beaudreau
Private Practice Dentist
4250 Washington Road
Augusta, GA 30809

Chester Douglass, Chairman
Department of Dental Care Administra-
tion
Harvard School of Dental Medicine
188 Longwood Avenue
Boston, MA 02115

Harold Frank, Vice President
Mithras Group
Management Consulting Company
P.O. Box 492
Buena Park, CA 91612

John Greene, Dean
School of Dentistry
University of California at San Francisco
Third and Parnassus Streets
San Francisco, CA 94143

Charles Jerge
Professor/Chairman
Department of Dentistry
School of Medicine
Wake Forest University
Director
Winston-Salem Dental Care Plan, Inc.
201 Charlois Boulevard
Winston-Salem, NC 27103

James Mercer
Private Practice Dentist
806 Akron Savings & Loan Building
Akron, OH 44308

Eugene Truono
Private Practice Dentist
2300 Pennsylvania Avenue
Wilmington, DE 19806
Trustee
American Dental Association

Stephen Wotman
Assistant Professor of Dentistry
School of Dentistry and Oral Surgery
Assistant Dean of Academic Affairs
School of Public Health
Columbia University
600 West 168th Street
New York, NY 10032

National Advisory Board cont.

Max Schoen
School of Dentistry
UCLA Center for the Health Sciences
Los Angeles, CA 90024

The Faculty and Staff of the Pennsylvania Experiment

Administration

D. Walter Cohen	
Patricia Cormier	Codirectors
Deborah Diserens	Coordinator of Curriculum and Evaluation
Peter Barnett	Director of Management Information Systems
Marguerita Bomba	Coordinator of Penn Faculty Plan and Computer Information Systems

Faculty

DIRECTORS:

Robert Tisot	Director of Model B
Daniel Casullo	Director of Model A and Advanced Dental Education Program
Uri Hangorsky	Director of Model A
Jeffrey Garber	Director of Model G

PRIMARY TEACHING FACULTY:

Model B
Norman Lurie
Robert Rose
Jeffrey Pearlman-Storch
Richard Subin
Gerald Weintraub
Vincent Trosiello
Leif Tronsted
Gunner Hasselgren
David Kerr
David Maltz
Annette Thomas

Bahman Sanikhatam
Christine McMahon, Dental Hygienist
Marie Carlisle, Dental Hygienist
Melanie Brakebill, Dental Hygiene Resident

Model A

Daniel Boston	Russell Phillips
Robert Emling	Louise Skarulis
Norman Kaplis	Woodrow Stevens
John Karabas	Denise Vezina
Richard Kaufman	Gerald Weger
Woodrow Kotch	Robert Wolf
Mark Lipkin	Irene Woodall
Barry Melman	Arthur Zack
Susan Muhler	Judith Zack, Dental Hygiene Resident

STAFF:

Model B

Helen Calvert	Ellen McCullough
Jane Caniz	Annette Muracco
Kathy Daniels	Geraldine Stouffer
Christine Kaufman	

Model A
Lisa Shildhorn
Sheryl Sinkow

DENTAL ASSISTANTS:

Model B

Kathy Cammeron	Patty Fells
Victoria Capewell	Deborah Levin-Sharpe
Carol Carey	Pam Lewis
Kelly Carey	Eva Nurenberg
Sharon Cohen	Bertha Rodgers
Venessa Dorsey	

Model A
Mary Hunt
Maureen Foelster
Norma Price

APPENDIX VI

Evaluation Steering Committee and Members of the Faculty Evaluation Team

Steering Committee
Peter Barnett   Daniel Boston
Robert DeRevere   Deborah Diserens
Patricia Cormier, Chair

Faculty Evaluation Teams
Preclinical Measures

1. Molar waxing (#3)   Daniel Boston
                                       David Maltz

2. Cl II Amalgam preparation (#29)   Basil Abrams
   Cl I   Amalgam preparation (#30)   Daniel Boston
   Cl III DFG preparation   Daniel Boston

3. Full dentures setup   Bal Goyal
                                       Heywood Kotch

4. Three unit bridge   Joseph Greenberg
                                       Robert Tisot

Clinical Measures

1. Diagnostic radiology   Robert Beideman
                                       Jerry Katz
                                       Denise Vezina

2. Local anesthesia technique   Jeffrey Garber
                                       Jerry Katz
                                       Denise Vezina

3. Junior treatment planning exam   Uri Hangorsky
                                       Daniel Maltz

4. Senior treatment planning exam   Daniel Boston
                                       Sol Rosenberg
                                       Richard Tobey

5. Periodontal therapy*   Uri Hangorsky
                                       Norman Stoller
                                       Denise Vezina

*This exam was not administered because of logistical difficulties in implementing this clinical exam as designed.

APPENDIX VII

Resident and Student Participants in the Pennsylvania Experiment (1979–1982)

MODEL A

Class of 1979
Stephen Grossman
Jack Keller
David Leibowitz
Bahman Sanikhetam

Class of 1980
Julie Barna
Marc Kipkin
Frederick Kwong
Fred Marra
Larry Schiff
Louise Skarulis-Celella

Class of 1981
Paul Brown
Willis Cardot
Carol Kirschenbaum
James Reese
John Weierbach
Craig Williams

Class of 1982
John Ford
Graeme Hudson
Mark Ruggerio
Mark Schwartz
Brian Shuman
Gregory Vergos

Class of 1983
Robert Bernstein
Steven Gilson
Joseph Keefer
Edward Kozinn
Venessa Morenzi
Thomas Oates
Jeffrey Sibner
Michael Yasner

Class of 1984
Donald Belcher
Mariya Brown
Bruce Freme
Brian Hogan
Jane Miller
Paul Pasternack
Jennifer Patterson

Class of 1985
Susan Braunstein
Steven Brisman
Rande Kaminsky
Bruce Kristiniak
David Silver
Jerry Statman
David Stermer

MODEL B

Class of 1979
Madalyn Ginsburg
Gary Rose
Robert Rose

Class of 1980
Shirley Brown
Marilyn MacLeod
Jeffrey Pearlman-Storch

Class of 1981
William Cheung
Jack Corn
Steven Locke
Jeffrey Rubin

Class of 1982
Gary Dworkin
Sara Chinn Karabasz
Robert Dworkin
Joseph Valenzi

Class of 1983
Meredith Bogert
Kenneth Carsto
Robert Dores
Thomas Gluck

Class of 1984
Clifford Capelli
Mitchell Cohen
Steven Isaccson
Stephen Kielceski
Suzanne Rubenstein

Class of 1985
Jeffrey Dorfman
Mark Dunayer
Paul Kost
Stewart Rauchman

Dental Hygiene Residency Questionnaire (1981–82)

Dental Student/Dental Resident Assessment

Please specify: _____ Dental Student, Graduation Date: 19___

_____ Dental Resident

Please identify your feelings regarding the following statements by circling appropriate number.

1. I believe that a DENTAL residency program is a valuable component of the education of a DENTAL student.

1	2	3	4	5
strongly disagree		no opinion		strongly agree

2. I believe that a DENTAL HYGIENE residency program is a valuable component of the education of a DENTAL HYGIENE student.

1	2	3	4	5
strongly disagree		no opinion		strongly agree

3. I believe that a DENTAL HYGIENE resident's presence in clinic would be of educational value for me.

1	2	3	4	5
strongly disagree		no opinion		strongly agree

4. I believe that my experience working with a DENTAL HYGIENE resident would influence my future decision to employ a dental hygienist.

1	2	3	4	5
strongly disagree		no opinion		strongly agree

5. At this point in my education, I am well aware of the level and variety of clinical skills and knowledge that a graduate dental hygienist possesses.

1	2	3	4	5
strongly disagree		no opinion		strongly agree

6. I believe that dental hygienists have clinical skills that are equal to dentists in the area of *non-surgical* periodontal therapy.

1	2	3	4	5
strongly disagree		no opinion		strongly agree

7. I believe that dental hygienists have skills that are equal to dentists in the area of basic emergency procedures.

1	2	3	4	5
strongly disagree *dentists* are more skilled		no opinion		strongly agree, dental hygienists are at least as skilled

8. I believe that dental hygienists are able to detect clinical extra- and/or intra-oral abnormalities, thereby assuring that patients will receive proper treatment and/or referral.

1	2	3	4	5
strongly disagree *dentists* are more skilled		no opinion		strongly agree, dental hygienists are at least as skilled

9. I believe that a dental hygienist who has completed a dental hygiene residency program would be a more knowledgeable and skilled clinician than a dental hygienist with one year of private practice experience.

1	2	3	4	5
strongly disagree		no opinion		strongly agree

10. I believe that a dental hygienist is a valuable member of a dental practice.

1	2	3	4	5
strongly disagree		no opinion		strongly agree

11. As of this date, my co-therapy* experience with a *dental hygiene student* would best be described as: (please circle appropriate letter)

   a. no experience

   b. limited experience (have provided co-therapy for 1–3 clinic patients)

   c. moderate experience (have provided co-therapy for 4–8 clinic patients)

   d. numerous experiences (have provided co-therapy for 9 or more clinic patients)

*Co-therapy is defined as that situation in which a patient's oral health needs are met through the *combined* efforts of a dental and dental hygiene student.

12. At the present time, my long-term professional goal is:

    _____ a.   to establish a General Dentistry private practice

    _____ b.   to work as a general dentist in an established dental practice/clinic

    _____ c.   to specialize in the following area:

        _____ 1) Pedodontics   _____ 5) Orthodontics

        _____ 2) Periodontics   _____ 6) Other: _____

        _____ 3) Endodontics

        _____ 4) Oral Surgery

    _____ d.   uncertain at this time

    _____ e.   other (please describe) _____

                        _____

APPENDIX IX

Junior Treatment Planning Examination

Following each case described below, *list the appropriate treatment(s)* (from the
treatment selections below) *in the correct sequence.* If an alternative treatment plan
is possible, indicate that sequence in a similar fashion. For each treatment selection
indicate the tooth or teeth involved.

KEY

a. Oral Hygiene Instruction
b. Scaling and Root Planing and Simple
     Prophylaxis
c. Periodontal Surgery
d. Orthodontic Therapy
e. Endodontic Therapy:
    1) Emergency pulp extirpation and
       opening the access
    2) Complete
f. Extraction
g. Amalgam Restoration(s)
h. C/B or onlay or inlay

i. Carious Excavation and
     temporization
j. Incision and Drainage
k. Occlusal Adjustment
l. Night Guard
m. No Treatment
n. Partial Denture
o. Reassess
p. Treatment for M.P.D.S.
q. Provisional
r. Refer (indicate specialty)
s. Hawley Therapy

EXAMPLE: A 40 year old woman with poor oral hygiene came into your office complaining of a toothache in tooth #13. A radiographic examination reveals
a large radiolucent area at the apex of the root of #13. A clinical exam
reveals an extensive carious lesion in this tooth. No other carious lesions
are present. The patient also reports grinding her teeth at night.

1. e (1 + 2) - #13
2. a - whole mouth
3. b - whole mouth   OR
4. q - #13
5. o - whole mouth
6. h - #13
7. l - whole mouth

1. e (1 + 2) - #3
2. a - whole mouth
3. b - whole mouth
4. h - #13
5. l - whole mouth

Code #: _____

1. Patient has poor oral hygiene, heavy calculous deposits, edematous bleeding gingival tissues, but no periodontal pockets. No other dental problems are present.

2. Patient has poor oral hygiene, heavy calculous deposits, edematous bleeding gingival tissues and no periodontal pockets are present. Radiographic interpretation examination reveals deep carious lesions in #30. No other problems are present.

3. A 60 year old patient comes to your office for a routine examination. The patient has no dental discomfort. During examination you discover #30 and #19 missing. (Patient reports having them extracted 30 years ago). No other dental problems are evident.

4. Patient bit on a plum pit about 2 weeks ago. He reports to your office with severe pain in #8. The tooth is very sensitive to percussion hot and cold. Radiographic examination reveals a vertical fracture extending from the occlusal surface down to the apex. No other dental problems are present.

5. A 35 year old female comes to your office. Examination reveals generalized Periodontitis (type III) and very small carious lesions in #30 and #29. No other dental problems are present.

6. A 20 year old male has combined painful periodontal-endodontic lesion on #13. Patient has otherwise healthy periodontium, but several other carious lesions are present in teeth #3, 4, 12, 14, and 19. Moderate amount of plaque and calculus are present, and there is mild gingival inflammation.

7. A 35 year old male presents to your office complaining of waking up in the morning with sore jaws. Your examination reveals numerous wear facets, left and right non-working prematurities. No other dental problems are present.

8. A 42 year old female has generalized Periodontitis (type II and III). Teeth #19 and 14 are in non-working and centric interference. There is fremitus in #5, 8, and 10. Tooth #30 has been extracted 20 years ago. No mesial drift has taken place; however, #4 has extruded 1.5 mm. Patient is interested in the best possible treatment.

9. History - A 65 year old man has just won the Pennsylvania Lottery. Now that he goes to Atlantic City a lot he has developed a complex about his appearance. He functions adequately. On clinical examination all molars are missing with a stable premolar to premolar occlusion. He is a periodontally resistant patient with only a slight marginal gingivitis.

10. History - A 20 year old patient presents with the following:

    1) Poor oral hygiene.
    2) Gross caries present in all teeth.
    3) Endodontic therapy needed on 16 of 32 teeth.
    4) Crowns needed on all teeth.
    5) No osseous involvement but marginal gingivae swollen and edematous and bleeds very easily. Deepest pocket 4 mm.
    6) Teeth with best prognosis #2, 6, 11, 15, 18, 21, 26, 27. They will need crowns but no endodontics.
    7) Patient is medically compromised with a past history of rheumatic fever.
    8) Patient has limited finances.

11. History - A 50 year old male presents with pain in the upper right quadrant; tinnitus and deviation of mandible to right hand side. On clinical examination there were the following findings:

1) Oral hygiene good.
2) No periodontal involvement.
3) No mobility patterns are present.
4) Many teeth show wear facets on guiding inclines.
5) X-rays reveal carious lesions on teeth #3, 4, 5. Caries has just penetrated dentine.
6) Radiographic findings of TMJ's are normal.

12. A patient presented with a main complaint that a bridge, which was constructed 8 years ago, is now mobile after patient bit on a hard object.

Clinical examination reveals:

1) Fracture of solder joint of bridge extending from teeth 29–31.
2) Patient has not seen a dentist for 8 years.
3) On comparing x-rays no change has taken place in osseous levels over an 8 year period.
4) Oral hygiene is poor.
5) Tooth #31 is tilted mesially. Osseous dips down from pontic area to mesial surface of tooth and is situated 3 mm. below cemento-enamel junction.
6) Pocket depth on mesial of #31 is 3 mm.

13. A very attractive 14 year old girl presented to your office with a discolored upper central incisor which was not possible to clean prophylactically. She wished to follow a career in modeling. The tooth was vital and had a normal x-ray appearance for a 14 year old girl. Oral hygiene was excellent and no caries present.

14. A very attractive 14 year old girl presented to your office with a discolored central incisor. She wished to follow a career in modeling. The tooth was non-vital. Pulp chamber was wide and no radiolucency present at apex. Oral hygiene was excellent and no caries present.

15. Patient presented with a main complaint of mobile teeth. On clinical examination the following was found:

1) 50% bone loss in all quadrants.
2) Vertical and horizontal bone loss.
3) Pockets of up to 7 mm. present in most areas.
4) Swollen, edematous, and inflamed gingivae.
5) Poor oral hygiene.
6) Mandibular first molar missing.
7) Mandibular second molars drifted mesially.
8) Maxillary first molars overerupted.
9) Maxillary anterior teeth drifted forward.
10) Mandibular anterior teeth drifted forward.
11) No caries.

16. Patient presented with pain in the lower right quadrant.
Findings: 1) Caries present in #28, 29, 30, 31.
Tooth #30 minimal occlusal caries.
Tooth #29 has an apical area of long standing and is non-vital.
Tooth #28 MOD cavity just penetrating dentine.
Tooth #31 a large distal carious lesion.
2) A large vertical osseous defect is present mesial to #28.
3) All teeth respond normally to percussion.
4) Oral hygiene is poor.
5) A generalized marginal gingivitis with only osseous lesion present in tooth #28 area.

What would be your priority order of treatment? Indicate order of teeth numbers in treatment.

17. A patient presents with pain in the upper right quadrant.

Findings: 1) Tooth #6 is vital, not painful to percussion and has no caries.

2) Tooth #5 is non-vital and has a fistula present. On placing an exploratory point, it points to the apex of #5. It is slightly painful to percussion and has a large MOD amalgam restoration present.

3) Tooth #4 has had endodontic therapy recently completed. The root canal treatment seems good and well condensed. An apical radiolucency is present. No previous x-rays are available.

4) Tooth #3 is non-vital, slightly painful to percussion. On x-ray it appears to have a large carious lesion which communicates with the pulp chamber.

What would be your priority order of treatment? Indicate order of teeth numbers in treatment.

18. Patient presents for check-up:

1) Full maxillary dentition.
2) 2nd premolar to 2nd premolar teeth present in mandible.
3) Molars extracted 6 years ago.
4) Slight overeruption of maxillary molars.
5) No caries or periodontal disease present.
6) Patient is 50 years old.

APPENDIX X

Senior Treatment Planning Examination
Case Report

A fifty-three-year-old female of heavy build presented with a chief complaint of wanting her teeth to be better looking, specifically, wanting her upper anteriors to "be longer." Esthetics is of prime importance to her, perhaps because she is an artist.

Her past dental history consisted of very irregular visits, as her husband was in the military, and she travelled and relocated often. She is uncomfortable discussing her dental history, as most of her visits were done on an emergency basis, and were all associated with pain. All of her missing teeth have been out for at least ten or fifteen years. She has never had Orthodontics, and is unaware of any tooth position changes, but she has been extremely unhappy with her upper front teeth and their positions since she was a teenager. Within the last two years, she has had all of her restorative/caries control done. A restoration was placed on every tooth in her mouth except the lower anteriors. She had been diagnosed at that time as having rampant caries, prior to having the operative dentistry. All endodontic therapy has been done for at least two years. She is not aware of any clenching, grinding or lip biting.

Her medical history is not contributory. A head and neck exam and a TMJ exam were all within normal limits. Although she has been overweight all her life, she has lost fifty pounds over the last two years under the care of a physician. At this time she is still a heavy person. She considers herself a very nervous person, and finds it difficult to discuss unpleasant topics, such as her diet, her dental care, and her dental experience.

Upon exam, there was generalized bleeding upon both superficial and deep probing. There was a discrepancy between IC and RC of 4 mm. (Vertical and 1 mm. horizontal, with the initial point of contact between teeth #2 and #31.) There is a sort of group function on the right, with no left non-working contacts. Left working movement has guidance on teeth #11 and #15, with no working contacts. Protrusive movements are guided by tooth #8. There is a minimal amount of fremitus on the upper anteriors.

She presents now with caries control having been done two years ago, and a need to have a better looking and of course functioning dentition. Money is not a consideration in developing a treatment plan. Due to her general improvement in caring for herself the previous two years, she seems to be truly motivated to care for her dentition, and to do whatever is necessary to create an improvement in her mouth.

Soon after her initial visits, she presented with swelling on the buccal of tooth #31. See the single radiograph of this tooth with gutta-percha point down the buccal furcation. This tooth tested non-vital and then probed 12 + on the direct buccal. Four weeks later, tooth #18 had the same type of swelling (see photo), and was also non-vital.

Patient Name _____

Chart No. _____

Student _____

UNIVERSITY of PENNSYLVANIA

SCHOOL OF DENTAL MEDICINE

COMPREHENSIVE DENTAL CHARTING

Perio Fac. Sig. _____

Rest Fac. Sig. _____

Date _____

	1	2	3	4	5	6	7	8	9	10	11	12	13	14	15	16

Facial

	1	2	3	4	5	6	7	8	9	10	11	12	13	14	15	16
Mobility		1				½			½	1						
Recession		3	4		2	1	1		1	1	1	2	3			
Mast. Mucosa		5	3		4	5	4	5	4	4	4	3	5	5	5	
Probing Depth Initial		436	584		323	324	414	423	324	424	423	323	325	547	726	
Probing Depth Reeval.																
Existing Rest.																
Defective Surface(s)																
Carious Surface(s)																

Palatal

	1	2	3	4	5	6	7	8	9	10	11	12	13	14	15	16
Recession			1								1	1	1-3	1		
Probing Depth Initial		624	534		423	324	414	325	323	323	423	325	524	527	646	
Probing Depth Reeval.																

Lingual

	1	2	3	4	5	6	7	8	9	10	11	12	13	14	15	16
Recession		2			3-1	2	1	1	1	1	1	2	134		2	
Mast. Mucosa		3			3	3	5	5	4	4	5	3	3		3	
Probing Depth Initial		335			224	424	325	312	223	324	323	323	523		233	
Probing Depth Reeval.																

Facial

	1	2	3	4	5	6	7	8	9	10	11	12	13	14	15	16
Mobility		1			1	½		1	1	1					1	
Recession		2			4-1	1	1	1	1	1	1	1	1-34		2	
Mast. Mucosa		0-2			1	3	2	3	3	4	3	3	3		4	
Probing Depth Initial		584			313	325	424	424	424	323	324	324	324		355	
Probing Depth Reeval.																
Existing Rest.																
Defective Surface(s)																
Carious Surface(s)																

	32	31	30	29	28	27	26	25	24	23	22	21	20	19	18	17

Part IA

INSTRUCTIONS: Your diagnosis should indicate to the examiners that you have a clear and complete understanding of the general disease state of this patient. Your diagnoses should be listed in order of the relative significance to this general disease state. Use as many lines as necessary and pair the etiology for each diagnosis on the corresponding line under etiology.

Diagnosis:

1. _____

2. _____

3. _____

4. _____

5. _____

6. _____

7. _____

8. _____

9. _____

10. _____

Etiology:

1. _____

2. _____

3. _____

4. _____

5. _____

6. _____

7. _____

8. _____

9. _____

10. _____

Part IB

List your sequence of treatment noting specific procedures and teeth or areas.

1. _____

2. _____

3. _____

4. _____

5. _____

6. _____

7. _____

8. _____

9. _____

10. _____

11. _____

12. _____

13. _____

14. _____

15. _____

16. _____

17. _____

18. _____

19. _____

20. _____

21. _____

22. _____

23. _____

24. _____

25. _____

26. _____

27. _____

28. _____

29. _____

30. _____

Part II

	Category	Condition	1	2	3	4	5	6	7	8	9	10	11	12	13	14	15	16	17	18	19	20	21	22	23	24	25	26	27	28	29	30	31	32
DIAGNOSIS		Gingivitis																																
	Perio-dontitis	Early																																
		Moderate																																
		Advanced																																
	Occlusal Trauma	Primary																																
		Secondary																																
	Endo	Perio/Endo																																
		Reversible Pulpitis																																
		Irreversible Pulpitis																																
		Caries																																
		Wear																																
TREATMENT	Perio Therapy	Extractions																																
		Phase I																																
		Phase II																																
	Occlusal Therapy	Selective Grinding																																
		Add-on Procedures																																
		Hawley Therapy																																
		Nite Guard Therapy																																
		Splinting																																
	Endo Therapy	Pulp Capping																																
		Total Obturation																																
		Single Tooth Restoration																																
		Fixed Prosthetics																																
		Removable Prosthetics																																
		Orthodontics																																

Part III

Questions: For each of the following questions choose the *one* best response from the available answers.

In questions 1–10 choose the tooth which has the *poorest* prognosis:
(Answer by circling the correct response)

1. a) #12	b) #20	c) #18
2. a) #20	b) #31	c) #18
3. a) #2	b) #20	c) #31
4. a) #2	b) #3	c) #18
5. a) #2	b) #14	c) #3
6. a) #2	b) #14	c) #15
7. a) #12	b) #20	c) #14
8. a) #2	b) #15	c) #20
9. a) #2	b) #11	c) #20
10. a) #3	b) #12	c) #31

Questions

11. Regarding definitive treatment for tooth #12 what finding would be the most important in making decisions for Phase II treatment at re-evaluation?

    a) None, I would have extracted #12
    b) Mobility
    c) Amount of sound tooth structure remaining
    d) Crown to root ratio

12. If tooth #6 tested vital, but was sensitive to percussion, your treatment would be:

    a) _____

    b) _____

c) _____

d) _____

13. Regarding tooth #31, what would be the most important initial finding regarding prognosis?

    a) None, I would extract
    b) Mobility
    c) Furcation Involvement
    d) Vitality

14. Regarding tooth #20, what is the most important finding regarding ultimate prognosis for this tooth?

    a) None, I would extract
    b) Lack of mobility
    c) Crown to root ratio
    d) Amount of sound tooth structure remaining

15. Regarding tooth #18, what is the most important finding regarding prognosis for this tooth?

    a) Vitality
    b) Periodontal abscess
    c) Furcation Involvement
    d) None, I would extract

16. Regarding tooth #15, what is the most important finding regarding prognosis for this tooth?

    a) Endodontic healing
    b) Furcation Involvement
    c) Root Proximity
    d) Lack of Mobility

17. Regarding tooth #3, what is the most important finding regarding prognosis for this tooth?

    a) Endodontic healing
    b) Furcation Involvement
    c) Root proximity
    d) Mobility

18. The decision to place a free gingival graft around tooth #20 depends most upon:

    a) The probing depth relative to the mucogingival junction
    b) The dimension of masticatory mucosa
    c) The placement of subgingival crown margin
    d) The dimension of exposed root from the free gingival margin to the CEJ

19. If the decision in treatment is to insert a Hawley Bite Plane, acceptable reasons for its placement would be what combination of the following?

    I. to increase the occluso-vertical dimension, primarily because of prior loss of vertical dimension
    II. to control parafunctional habits
    III. posterior eruption
    IV. to increase the occluso-vertical dimension, primarily for restorative reasons

V. to establish the retruded contact position
   a) II, III, V
   b) II, III
   c) II, IV, V
   d) II, V
   e) I, II, IV

20. If at periodontal re-evaluation, soft tissue consistency appears within normal limits, and the pocket depths in the mandibular left quadrant are as shown:

Tooth #	24	23	22	21	20	19
B	212	212	214	512	213	323
L	212	212	215	412	213	323

Your treatment would be:

a) Gingivectomy
b) Apical positioned flap with osseous resective procedures
c) Apical positioned flap without osseous resective procedures
d) Open curettage with osseous resective procedures
e) None of the above

For the next questions assume you are limited in treating this case and *have to remove teeth.*

A. Which one tooth of the three in each question would you extract; if you *had* to extract one?

   21. (a) 12   (b) 18   (c) 20
   22. (a) 18   (b) 20   (c) 31
   23. (a)   3   (b) 18   (c) 31
   24. (a) 15   (b) 18   (c) 31
   25. (a)   3   (b) 12   (c) 15

B. Which one tooth of these below would you consider most important to retain in restoring the case with partials?

   26. (a)   2   (b) 20   (c) 31
   27. (a)   3   (b) 12   (c) 13
   28. (a)   2   (b)   5   (c) 15
   29. (a) 15   (b) 18   (c) 20
   30. (a)   5   (b)   6   (c) 13

Part IV

1. Now that you have completed Part III of the exam please list any changes that you would now make in Diagnosis, Etiology, and/or Treatment and your reasons why.

2. Are there any aspects of the treatment which you would refer out? If so, please indicate which steps and *indicate the reason why.*

Index

Figures and tables are indicated by "f" or "t" following the page number.

215